The Future of Health

How Digital Technology Will Make Care Accessible, Sustainable, and Human

ROBERTO ASCIONE

WILEY

Published by John Wiley & Sons, Inc., Hoboken, New Jersey.
Published simultaneously in Canada.

For general information on our other products and services or for technical support, please contact our Customer Care Department within the United States at (800) 762-2974, outside the United States at (317) 572-3993 or fax (317) 572-4002.

Wiley also publishes its books in a variety of electronic formats. Some content that appears in print may not be available in electronic formats. For more information about Wiley products, visit our web site at www.wiley.com.

Library of Congress Cataloging-in-Publication Data

Names: Ascione, Roberto, author.
Title: The future of health: how digital technology will make care accessible,
   sustainable, and human / Roberto Ascione.
Other titles: Futuro della salute. English
Description: Hoboken, New Jersey : Wiley, [2022] | Translation of Il futuro
   della salute / Roberto Ascione. Milano : Ulrico Hoepli editore, 2018. |
   Includes bibliographical references and index.
Identifiers: LCCN 2021034635 (print) | LCCN 2021034636 (ebook) | ISBN
   9781119797258 (cloth) | ISBN 9781119797326 (Adobe PDF) | ISBN
   9781119797319 (ePub)
Subjects: MESH: Medical Informatics | Digital Technology | Delivery of
   Health Care—trends | Biomedical Technology—trends | United States |
   Europe
Classification: LCC R855.3 (print) | LCC R855.3 (ebook) | NLM W 26.5 |
   DDC 610.285—dc23
LC record available at https://lccn.loc.gov/2021034635
LC ebook record available at https://lccn.loc.gov/2021034636

Cover image: © Alfredo De Simone, Creative Director at Healthware Group
Cover design: Wiley

SKY10030303_100521

To my father,
doctor for the people and
maestro for life

Contents

Preface   xi

PART I   **Digital Reflections**   **1**

CHAPTER 1 Devices, Sensors, and Signals   3
              From Wearables to Ingestibles—Toward the
              Invisibility of Digital Health   4
              Roberto's View   5
              Apple Watch   6
              Empatica   8
              Proteus Digital Health   8
              Qardio   9
              Thync   10
              Note   14

CHAPTER 2 Data Science and Artificial Intelligence   15
              Using Big Data to Do Mass Screening
              and Prevention   16
              Roberto's View   18
              Conversa Health   19
              One Drop   20
              Sensely.com   21
              SkinVision   23
              Notes   27

CHAPTER 3 Evolution of the Computer-Human Interfaces
              in Health Care   29
              Roberto's View   32
              Alexa and Echo   33

Babylon and Healthily   34
HoloLens   36
MindMaze   37
Pepper Robot   37
Psious   38
PatchAi   39
Notes   39

CHAPTER 4   Telemedicine and Remote Monitoring   41
How Telemedicine Will Change Our Lives   42
Covid-19: The Tipping Point of Telehealth   44
Roberto's View   44
Omada Health   45
Sano   46
Teladoc Health   46
TytoCare   47
VitalConnect   48
Notes   51

CHAPTER 5   Digital Health Enabling Platforms   53
Platforms for Connecting Doctors and Patients,
Remote Monitoring Systems, and Management
of Their Therapies   54
Roberto's Vision   56
Altibbi   57
Apple Health   58
Cohealo   59
DocDoc   60
Doctolib   60
hi.health   61
Livongo   61
Paginemediche   62
Notes   69

CHAPTER 6   Digital Therapeutics   71
Roberto's Vision   74
Akili   76

	Amicomed	77
	Click Therapeutics	78
	Ginger.io	79
	Kaia Health	79
	Voluntis	80
	Notes	83
CHAPTER 7	Personal Genomics	85
	From Mendel to Portable DNA Mapping Machines	86
	Roberto's Vision	88
	23andMe	90
	Deep Genomics	91
	Flatiron Health	92
	Human Longevity	93
	Sophia Genetics	94
	Cellarity	94
	Notes	97
CHAPTER 8	Open Innovation and Partnerships	99
	How Companies Are Moving: The Speed and Intuition of Smaller Companies	100
	Roberto's Vision	101
	AlmirallShare and Digital Garden	103
	Bayer G4A	104
	Frontiers Health	104
	Healthware Labs and Healthware Life Hub	105
	HealthXL	106
	Johnson & Johnson Innovation Labs (JLABS)	107
	Novartis Biome	107
	Open Accelerator	107
	Patients' Digital Health Awards	108
	Pfizer Healthcare Hubs	108
	Roche HealthBuilders	109
	StartUp Health	109
	Vertical	110
	Notes	119

CHAPTER 9 Lifestyle as Medicine   121
From Self-Empowerment to Lifestyle as Medicine   122
Roberto's Vision   123
Headspace   125
HealthTunes   126
Noom   127
Sleepio   127
Pioppi Protocol   128
YourCoach.health   128

PART II   **Human Reflections**   **131**

CHAPTER 10 The New Physicians and Patients   135
An Ever-Increasing Pressure   136
Will Doctors Disappear?   138
Necessary Scientific Validation   139
Patients as Health-Care Consumers   140

CHAPTER 11 Old versus New   141
A Necessary Adaptation   142
New Training   143
A Collective Effort Is Needed   144
Note   145

CHAPTER 12 Trust versus Fear   147
The Horizon Opening Before Us   148
Double face medal   149

CHAPTER 13 Exponential versus Incremental   151
A Financial Revolution Too   152
Digital Health-Care Investments around the World   154
A Glance toward the Future   159
Notes   159

Conclusions   A Radical Shift **161**

Appendix 175

About the Author 177

About Healthware 179

Acknowledgments 181

Index 183

Preface

I have been involved in medicine and digital technologies for over 25 years.

I trained as a doctor but never became one because I was also passionate about computer science and torn between these two elements: programming and medicine. I realized that everything in health care was largely analog, and still is in many ways. I started writing my own software using MIT's Logo programming language in middle school, and ever since I had been fascinated by the idea that, using computer science, you could write software to manage practically any problem. It was an intuition that time has confirmed!

I started to realize that health care and computer science had something in common: code! Both DNA and software programming languages were code, so I had the idea to combine these two passions of mine and to deal with digital technology and medicine. I realized very early on that there was no existing role for this, and I didn't know of a single company considering this dual discipline. Everyone advised me against entering this nonexistent field, but by the time I was almost a doctor, I decided to follow my instincts and founded a company called Healthware, so named because it was at the intersection of health care and software. The initial idea was very simple: to create software for medicine by providing better treatment tools for doctors, which resulted in better treatment for patients.

What was my motivation?

If I had been a doctor, even a very good one, I would have had a limited impact on a few thousand people. By producing software for the health-care world, the impact could be much greater. Healthware was born of this idea. It started to grow quite rapidly during the first years—and we are still here talking about it 25 years later.

Healthware was founded in southern Italy and is now present in various parts of the world. However, we are not here to talk about Healthware, but rather about what we help to cultivate: the development of digital health to improve lives.

Let's start with a few concepts that may certainly seem obvious, but are not as simple as they appear.

Digital technology is ubiquitous, and many aspects of our individual lives are already largely linked to digital platforms for service, communication, or social sharing. These dimensions of daily life are now totally linked to these systems and technologies, which has effects on an entire series of processes: economic, productive, psychological, behavioral, and much more. This phenomenon has also occurred in the health sector, where it has obviously changed a lot of things over the past few years. We have become accustomed to enjoying certain platform services that have profoundly transformed various sectors, from the hotel industry to the music industry. We have also become both producers and consumers at the same time. Let's think about music: not only is it no longer bought and sold as it was before, but because of the way it is consumed, it is no longer produced in the same way. Musicians don't create albums with two hits and a B-side anymore. (Remember long-playing albums with 10-songs?). Now consumers buy one song at a time, so artists must produce 10 good songs if they want ten hits. As these patterns permeate various industries, they change them dramatically. All this combined is not just a marginal change, but a radical transformation of health that has an even greater scope than that of music or travel.

I feel this change, and the challenge it underlies, deep down. When these radical transformations come, a moment of change occurs, with a before and an after. In the aftermath, you can find yourself on the side of companies, even very important ones, that had access to these innovations at the right time, but did not follow them, such companies were overwhelmed. The alternative is to be on the side of companies that grasped these transformations, perhaps starting from scratch, and today find themselves playing a role that simply didn't exist before. I believe that health care has entered this zone of radical transformation and what we are witnessing is incomparable to anything we have known in the last 40 to 50 years.

I'll make a few preliminary considerations to frame the world in which we are moving, and consequently correlate them to the digital development taking place in the health sector. Precisely to anticipate needs and trends, it is increasingly common for analysts to study the so-called megatrends (i.e., forecasts of the medium- to long-term trends that will emerge).

Viewing the forecasts for the next 15 years (i.e., the megatrends related to 2030), we discover some things that will have a very strong impact. Meanwhile, demographers estimate that the world's population will reach 8.6 billion people by 2030, compared to 7.86 billion in 2021. That is a monstrous figure that will have economic, industrial, nutritional, and political impacts. First of all, think of the life expectancy increase and consequent health problems linked to an aging population, and the subsequent need to organize the related caregiving mechanisms. And managing the health of 8.6 billion people will cost significantly more than what's required for 7.8 billion people; an increase that will make the current form and level of care unsustainable. All of this will turn into a giant acceleration element of transformation.

Parallel to global population growth, as of today, 5 billion people have internet access—an increase of 1 billion over 2017. In addition, the new mobile broadband, 5G, will increasingly bring omnipresent connectivity even to territories lacking infrastructure, facilitating, for example, access to schooling for children in remote regions of Africa and Asia.

Of course, this phenomenon will also increasingly enable access to telemedicine and even robotic telesurgery. (The first practical demonstrations of 5G applications in this area date back to 2019, when a Chinese neurosurgeon was able to operate on a patient suffering from Parkinson's disease 3,000 kilometers away.)

The result of this health transformation, thanks to technology, is an increasingly better prepared and better cared-for population. More connectivity means an ever-increasing knowledge of health digitization, and consequently, an increasing demand for certain services. In a word, it will ensure greater and, subsequently, universal access to care. It is a real revolution, and as such, unstoppable, because everything is moving on an exponential scale and time frame, especially if we pause to reflect on concepts such as the speed and cost of technology availability, diffusion, and habits of digital culture.

We might think about going even further, imagining leveraging technology, including widespread connectivity and continuous and integrated data collection, and placing the person at the center of the social health system and the care pathway. The great added value would be that individuals could monitor their own state of health or that of loved ones, and access dedicated digital services at any time, from anywhere. Furthermore, by cross-referencing our personal genetic information (we know genetic screening will be increasingly available to everyone) with the information in our digital health profile (all the data we actively or passively collect about our health), we will be able to make accurate predictions about the probability of developing a disease before it happens and implement countermeasures.

The concept of digital health goes beyond telemedicine and the collection of large amounts of data; it includes, in fact, all the digital innovations that fuel this paradigm shift in a disruptive way. I am referring to wearables and integrated sensors, predictive analytics systems based on artificial intelligence (AI), and machine learning that is applicable to virtually every area of health, digital therapies, and much more.

In part this is what has already happened during the pandemic, with digital solutions that have served to support patients, caregivers, and health professionals in adherence to therapies, or in the diagnosis and treatment of certain chronic conditions, thus beginning to shift the focus from therapy (cure) to the care of people (care).

PART I

Digital Reflections

Digital technologies are part of our life flow. We use them to study and work, to connect with people, and also to do our grocery shopping, entertain ourselves, and find love. Health is not an exception albeit it is a much more recent discovery.

Through the usage of social media and other digital platforms we constantly create and nurture our digital footprint, often passively or without recognizing it. Despite this, many of these information or data points are relevant for our own health, even if we are not yet leveraging them to the fullest.

Cheaper, smaller, faster computers together with ever-evolving form factors from laptop to wearable and beyond have been enabling all-new use cases and practices, showing us that it is possible to quantify our health experiences. Over time, this has inspired a continuous evolution of personal medical devices, adding an objective and quantitative dimension to health and medicine that was completely unheard of only 10 years ago.

Novel technologies also unlocked access to the human genome, popularizing a practice which, only few years back, was extremely expensive and available only to academia and primary research. In other words, for a few hundred dollars we can get our full genome mapping, and for even less we can investigate our genetic set-up regarding specific areas or conditions.

This unprecedented amount of data, originated both by digital and genetic signals, needed completely new strategies and computer-science solutions, which we often refer to as AI, to make sense of them.

AI and more appropriately data science are not only giving order to this vast amount of data but are also allowing us to correlate it with medical observations, unveiling connections and cause–effect implications which, in certain cases, we did not even imagine in the past.

Once these connections are scientifically proven, we can start to introduce them into the medical practice, often allowing for predictions of future evolution of certain disease states even before such a disease would develop.

Most of these innovations are coming from what we now identify as digital health startups, brave teams of young innovators and experienced professionals, often including doctors and other health-care professionals, engineers, designers, and patients, who are not afraid to challenge the status quo of health care and the implied inaccessibility, inconvenience, and uncertainty that are huge problems in the industry. This movement has been increasingly fueled by venture capital investments, which have been propelling this sector since 2011 and further accelerated through the Covid-19 pandemic of 2020.

All of this is having a profound impact on health care and its determinates, including health literacy, access to care, ability to connect to the right health-care resources, cost of diagnoses and therapies, prevention strategies, and more.

The first section of this book will review the most important technology innovations and provide examples of startups using them to foster this radical transformation of health care as we know it.

Devices, Sensors, and Signals

From Wearables to Ingestibles—Toward the Invisibility of Digital Health

Perhaps the most striking case of a radical health-care transformation, from a media point of view, was the launch of the Apple Watch on September 9, 2014. In reality, the market for wearables and network-connected devices had already been established for some time, especially in the sport sector: smart bracelets that calculated the number of steps taken in a day, the calories consumed, the amount and quality of sleep, and a whole host of other data were already on the market well before Apple launched itself into the enterprise.

According to *Forbes*, the wearables market was worth $27.9 billion in 2019 and is estimated to reach $74.03 billion in 2025. The sector includes smartwatches, fitness trackers, wristbands, and all those wearables that control physical activity or other vital parameters. And this value, according to estimates, is bound to grow even more. Technological developments have been leading to a progressive miniaturization of the components, to such an extent that nanotechnology-based devices are already available in the healthcare field. (Nanotechnology refers to technological structures smaller than one nanometer, one billionth of a meter.) This advance allows for more precise and less invasive diagnostic analysis, or tools that can even carry out intervention therapies at the molecular level. As is often the case in the field of technology, while the instruments become more powerful and complex, their cost of production is constantly decreasing, making the various devices accessible to an ever-widening range of consumers. The great ductility of the materials produced makes it possible to integrate processors and sensors into nearly every object of everyday use: shoes, T-shirts, appliances, toys, balls, racquets—everything can be made smart and connected at the cost of just a few dollars. And in the health field? The adoption of digital devices is a natural and inevitable process. The possibility of remotely monitoring the various devices connected to the network, the miniaturization of the components, and the evolution of the various sensors to become increasingly precise and reliable, allow the creation of wearables that can track diverse vital parameters without being uncomfortable for the wearer. This reduces (or even excludes) the need for a patient to go to the hospital or to visit a health-care professional for ongoing tests for conditions that need constant monitoring. For example, a health-care professional can monitor a patient's health remotely by accessing, in real time, data transmitted by a pacemaker connected to his or her mobile phone. The possible variations are endless.

Among the first pioneering therapies based on wearable technology, we remember the solution developed by Proteus Digital Health: a pill with a built-in micro-sensor. Once the pill is swallowed, the microcircuit sends signals to a patch on the patient's skin, which in turn communicates with the dedicated app on the patient's smartphone.

Roberto's View

We have gone from carrying with us very heavy and very expensive laptops with minimal computing power by today's standards, to using handheld computers, smartphones, tablets, and wearables. The process continues with the miniaturization and low cost of these devices reaching a point at which they are even *ingestible*. The widespread dissemination of these instruments among the public makes it possible to gather a quantity of information that was previously impossible. And this information, as it accumulates and we learn how to process it and act consequentially, begins to take on an ever-higher value from the standpoint of health care. We are, therefore, witnessing a widespread use of tracking instruments, created in the wellness or sports world, that are finding new applications in other areas. Indeed, ever-more-powerful algorithms analyze vast amounts of data, and correlations between this data and the most common pathologies are being discovered. On this basis, a new category of markers, called *digital biomarkers*, has been created. These are beginning to be examined in exactly the same way that normal blood tests are examined. In other words, researchers begin to monitor signals that may be related to particular disorders and then validate them with the idea of having markers that can be used to identify particular pathologies digitally in the future. For example, for attention disorders and Alzheimer's disease, applications of this type already exist and are currently undergoing clinical trials. Of course, in order to transform a normal process, we must identify a digital marker that is actually valid and scientifically sustainable. For example, there is a trial that is examining whether a certain type of continuous electrocardiogram (ECG), made with very low-cost sensors that could be incorporated into T-shirts, is predictive of major cardiac events, such as heart attacks. Let's imagine that this becomes possible and that, in the next few years, the sensors are so inexpensive that any T-shirt can make this kind of prediction. As a result, the management of a critical health event such as a heart attack (which requires immediate intervention in the place where it occurs) could be achieved with a routine operation such as an angioplasty.

Such sensors would be able to signal the likelihood of developing a certain pathology, and thus prompt the individual to schedule a specialist visit. This would completely change the management and treatment of a pathology as we imagine it today. Important transformations are taking place regarding the management of the personal data of each one of us: just think of the latest versions of the iOS and Android operating systems, in which real computerized medical records dedicated to the consumer/patient have been introduced. The symptom journal is a feature already embedded in operating systems that allows users to collect a large amount of information in a structured and processable way. A considerable number of clinical trials already have access to a much larger database than before. This data has been generated by participants thanks to the presence of these integrated applications in most smartphones.

Apple Watch

Apple Watch was certainly not the first instrument on the market among the wearables. However, it has been one of the cornerstones in the health-care revolution. Through not only its built-in functions, but also scenarios it makes possible, it has proposed itself as a common interface to numerous health apps that can communicate with it. This is why the Apple Watch has turned out to be a very important instrument for increasing a patient's adherence to their health-care program. In fact, specific apps can send alerts to remind a person to take a particular medicine, or they can use the Apple Watch's sensor network to make predictions about certain pathologies and recommend specific health checks.

Since 2019, Apple Watch users can take part in the three medical studies launched by the health-care giant in collaboration with leading academic and research institutes, to monitor women's health, investigate the correlation between heart rate and mobility signals, and assess the impact that the daily exposure to sound has on hearing.

In the same year, the ECG function was made available to all the users of the Apple Watch Series 4. The ECG app makes it possible to record the user's heart rate and rhythm using an electric heart sensor, and then to check the recording for the presence of atrial fibrillation (AF). The ability of the app to accurately classify an ECG recording as AF was tested in a clinical trial involving about 600 subjects. The app had a 98.3 percent sensitivity in the classification of atrial fibrillation, and a 99.6 percent specificity in the classification of the normal sinus rhythm.

An important step in Apple's push to market its Apple Watch as a health and fitness device is represented by the agreements it has struck with insurance companies such as Aetna, United Healthcare, and Devoted Health, which are subsidizing the cost of the device for their policyholders.

Apple is joining forces with researchers to conduct three health studies that include using Apple Watch to explore how blood oxygen levels can be used in future health applications. This year, Apple will collaborate with the University of California, Irvine, and Anthem to examine how longitudinal measurements of blood oxygen and other physiological signals can help manage and control asthma.

Separately, Apple will work closely with investigators at the Ted Rogers Centre for Heart Research and the Peter Munk Cardiac Centre at the University Health Network, one of the largest health research organizations in North America, to better understand how blood oxygen measurements and other Apple Watch metrics can help with the management of heart failure. Finally, investigators with the Seattle Flu Study at the Brotman Baty Institute for Precision Medicine and faculty from the University of Washington School of Medicine will seek to learn how Apple Watch can detect signals related to heart rate and blood oxygen, which could serve as early signs of respiratory conditions like influenza and Covid-19.[1]

Empatica

Empatica Inc., a spin-off of MIT's Media Lab, with offices in Cambridge and Milan, has built a smartwatch based on an advanced machine learning algorithm. It is capable of identifying seizures and sending alerts to the caregivers, recording sleep and rest data, and detecting electrodermal activity (EDA). EDA allows researchers to quantify physiological changes in the sympathetic nervous system, also known as the fight-or-flight response. It is the first device linked to a neurological condition that has been approved by the FDA.

Certified in Europe and the United States, Empatica's Embrace 2 is a device for adults and children over the age of 6. In a multisite clinical trial, 135 patients diagnosed with epilepsy were admitted to high-level monitoring units for continuous monitoring of level IV epilepsy. There, video electroencephalography (EEG) was used to monitor their brain activity. Simultaneously, they wore an Empatica device. In 272 days, 6,530 hours of data were recorded, including 40 generalized tonic-clonic seizures. Embrace's algorithm has been shown to detect 100 percent of the seizures.

Proteus Digital Health

Proteus Digital Health, an American company founded in 2001 with headquarters in Redwood City, California, had set itself an ambitious goal: to design and create "digital" drugs. To achieve this, it concentrated on developing products, services, and data systems based on the integration of ingestible drugs and cloud computing. In early 2017, in collaboration with Otsuka Pharmaceutical, Proteus developed a pill called Abilify MyCite, which incorporates a microsensor containing copper, silicon, and magnesium. The sensor is about the size of a grain of sand and is seamlessly eliminated through the digestive track. It was the first digital pill to receive the approval of the Food and Drug Administration (FDA), the American authority that regulates new drugs and medical treatments. Abilify MyCite is an antipsychotic product based on aripiprazole, a molecule used in the treatment of bipolar disorders and schizophrenia. The digital version developed by Proteus contains a sensor activated by gastric acids in the stomach that sends a message to a patch applied to the patient's skin. The message is in turn sent to a smartphone. This data can be accessed, with consent, by the patient's health-care professional, family members, or even by friends. It is no coincidence that the first application of the digital pill concerns mental illness, where failure to adhere to treatment is often a serious problem. According to experts, non-adherence to prescribed treatments (i.e., not taking medicines or not taking the right amount) would cost, in the United States alone, between $100 and $300 billion per year.

Despite the huge need for adherence solutions and Proteus's level of innovation, this solution never scaled, probably because it was ahead of its time in the context of the health-care industry. In mid-2020 Otsuka ended up acquiring Proteus, so perhaps full integration with a pharmaceutical company will allow this technology to be more broadly available to patients and doctors.

Qardio

Qardio is a wireless tool for detecting systolic and diastolic blood pressure, heart rate, and irregular heartbeats. Based on that alone, it would seem to share quite a lot with other devices on the market. What makes Qardio a very useful and interesting instrument for those who have heart problems (or for those who want to monitor their activities to monitor or prevent certain cardio pathologies) is the integration of the Qardio app with Apple Health and Apple Watch. This makes it possible to have an extremely easy and intuitive overview of the data. It also makes it possible to share the data automatically with friends and family or send them directly to a health-care professional via email. In particular, this latest integration is an important shortcut in the supply chain of doctor-patient communication, and it allows the information process to become more efficient. Both of these aspects benefit the health of the Qardio user. All the measurements recorded by the device are automatically stored in a special cloud space and made available for consultation through easy-to-read charts and tables. In this way, one always has an up-to-date history of measurements, anomalies, and trends related to moments of cardiac stress.

Thync

Thync is a small device aimed at reducing anxiety and ensuring a pleasant sleep. It rests on the neck and is managed via a smartphone app, giving users a choice between one of two programs. In the United States, much importance is given to the dangers of stress. According to studies of the American Psychological Association, it is in our times that the highest number of anxious states has been recorded in the history of the American population. Thync was developed by a team of neuroscientists at the Massachusetts Institute of Technology (MIT) and it went through five years of trials and thousands of test sessions. The instrument uses electrostimulation to alter the state of the brain and help the users relieve stress and anxiety without necessarily resorting to the use of anxiolytic drugs. The triangular device should be placed on the neck, at the back of the head, or on the forehead, and then activated: Thync, through small electric discharges, interacts with the nervous system, helping the wearer to recover his or her psychophysical balance for an improvement in health. "Neurostimulation is based on the link between the nerves located in the back of the neck and two areas of the brain, which affect stress and sleep" explains Isy Goldwasser, CEO of the company. But researchers want to push Thync beyond the boundaries of its original purpose, toward even more ambitious goals. They began with the assumption that the scientific literature is increasingly highlighting the important role that the nervous system plays in regulating the immune response in diseases such as psoriasis, lupus, inflammatory bowel disease (IBD), and rheumatoid arthritis. This led, in 2017, to the first trial of Thync in the treatment of psoriasis.

In the blind study, 28 subjects followed a treatment program (or a placebo program) every day for 10 minutes over the course of four weeks. After this time, 15 of the 18 subjects in the treatment group (83 percent of the total) reported at least a 50 percent reduction in the symptoms of psoriasis while 6 out of 18 subjects showed a reduction of more than 75 percent of these symptoms. In comparison, only 2 out of 10 subjects in the control group with the placebo program showed a 50 percent reduction in symptoms and no one had improvement of 75 percent ($p = 0.0005$). Thync is currently conducting clinical trials to further validate noninvasive modulation as a treatment for plaque psoriasis.

Guest Perspectives

MATTEO LAI
CEO, Emaptica

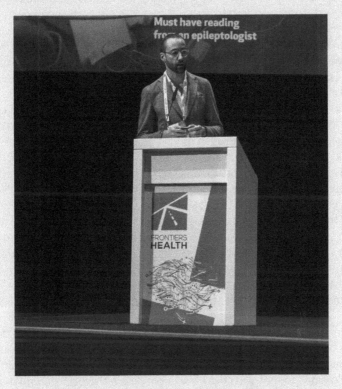

Matteo Lai speaking at Frontiers Health 2018
Credit: Frontiers Health

The reason why we started Empatica, together with Simone, Roz, and Maurizio, my co-founders, was to create technology and products that help people manage their health.

Our brains did not evolve fast enough to cope with the complexity of the modern world. That is something we see every day, with people struggling with mental health, or suffering from chronic conditions that are completely preventable. Our objective was very ambitious: we imagined a world where

(Continues)

(Continued)

the extreme complexity of human behavior and health is mapped and provided to each person, to get help and recommendations while navigating daily life. We imagined we would be building predictive analytics models, biomarkers that could monitor people's health automatically and unobtrusively. We knew it was going to be a long journey, but we had some principles in mind: these products would have to be based on cutting-edge science and technology. They would have to be beautiful and easy to use. They would empower each person and not become a system of surveillance to control them. So, we started building devices and algorithms to monitor real-time vital signs and autonomic nervous system activity.

Today, these products are used by thousands of researchers in the best hospitals and universities globally. They also support some of the world's largest pharmaceutical companies to run better clinical trials remotely. We then decided to help patients directly, with our first consumer product. In 2018, we introduced Embrace2, the first smartwatch to be cleared by FDA in neurology, designed to detect seizures for people living with epilepsy, providing lifesaving help to patients.

In the same year, we started developing an algorithm that would detect influenza infections. Following the outbreak of the Covid-19 pandemic we shifted the algorithm capabilities so that it could also detect the presence of SARS-CoV-2. With our wearables, it became the first wrist-worn solution to receive the European CE mark for Covid-19 detection, letting people know every morning if they should self-isolate and seek additional help, before they started feeling unwell.

We maintain our philosophy of building a revolutionary medical device with a beautiful design, expanding on our idea of applying AI to build biomarkers to support people's health. What if a cute little watch could predict migraines so that you could take a pill before the pain starts? What if it could understand if you are at risk of encountering a time of low mood or a depressive episode, providing you with help to avoid that altogether? What if you could understand what the most stressful events in your daily life are, empowering you and your partner with better insights? What if the watch could know you are getting ill before you know it?

This is not science fiction: we are currently running multiple clinical studies on these exact applications, with some of the leading experts in the world, to bring it from research to a real product. And it is very exciting to imagine how a better understanding of ourselves could help us live a better life.

SHANTI RAMAKRISHNAN
CEO eDevice

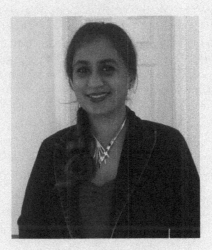

Shanti Ramakrishnan
Credit: Shanti Ramakrishnan

The healthcare industry has always been notorious for moving at a glacial pace and debates about the efficacy, efficiency, and access to care are unending. However, a global pandemic like Covid-19 provoked a sudden sea change. Various models of health-care delivery like virtual care, connected care, telemedicine, telehealth, and so on, which were languishing for decades with poor adoption rates became the modus operandi—and they have sustaining power.

Our company swiftly transformed and responded to this context switch. Specifically, we reoriented our company's mission of *connectivity that cares* to become a platform company that offers simplicity in obtaining health care and efficiency in providing it. Through orchestration and partnerships with medical sensors and device manufacturers; clinical specialists at hospitals; clinics; doctor's offices; patients and consumers; user experience (UX) experts; and with organic investments, we recreated and re-launched HealthGo, a platform that connects patients and health-care providers to enable connected care. Designed for simplicity, HealthGo can equally serve primary and routine care for specialized chronic conditions with predictive smart algorithms to prevent costly treatment.

(Continues)

(*Continued*)

> Various forms of signals (scientific, technical, market, etc.) have existed since time immemorial. Capturing and processing many signals, most often in real-time, via sensors, devices, or other input mechanisms is continuous and relentless. With ubiquitous and always-on connections, one can drown in data. In order to make a lasting impact, we learned that simplicity is complex and complicated. The challenge of discerning signals from noise is real, but many technical and business challenges can benefit from past context switches and successful reinvention.

Note

1. Apple. "Apple Watch Series 6 delivers breakthrough wellness and fitness capabilities," press release, September 15, 2020. Available at: https://www.apple.com/newsroom/2020/09/apple-watch-series-6-delivers-breakthrough-wellness-and-fitness-capabilities/.

CHAPTER 2

Data Science and Artificial Intelligence

Using Big Data to Do Mass Screening and Prevention

Verum scire est scire per causas, true knowledge is a knowledge of the causes. This was written by Thomas Aquinas, taking up one of the cornerstones of Aristotelian philosophy. It is in this belief—pin the discovery of the cause of a phenomenon—that the scientific method is oriented. Let it be understood, it still does this, but big data analysis has short-circuited this procedure. The science of big data causes, in the opinion of many, a decisive paradigm shift away from the past, based on a style of scientific reasoning that is totally different from what it once was. It is possible to draw a linear path in the history of science: an almost exclusively empirical approach consisting of the mere observation and description of natural phenomena followed the theoretical approach, which was based on the construction of models and the overall explanation of phenomena through general laws. The last phase, born a few decades ago, is the computational phase, which has as its cornerstone the simulation of complex phenomena through computerized models. Along this line, data-driven science stands as a new phase, a new piece of the jigsaw puzzle, a new milestone where experiment, theory, and data processing are synthesized in statistics. The use of big data to do mass screening and prevention is based on the identification of patterns, regularities, cyclical repetitions, and large-scale correlations that make it possible to process a prediction of what will be most likely to be found in the real world in similar contexts. In the science of health care, this predictive technique is made possible both by the enormous advances in the technology and biomedical fields in recent years (and the acceleration in this direction is astounding) and by access to an enormous amount of data, something that was unthinkable until recently. Suffice it to say that we are now able to synthesize an impressive amount of information from various sources. The amount is in the range of several petabytes (one petabyte corresponds to 1,000,000 gigabytes). The computer that allowed the Apollo 11 lunar module to land had a memory in the range of 104 bytes, so just this one comparison should be enough to understand the extent of the acceleration that has taken place in the field of data processing. However, there are some obvious critical issues in this methodology as it is applied to health. The first obstacle is the objective difficulty in governing this huge mass of data, especially when it is used and applied differently from the initial purpose of their collection. Then there is, of course, an obstacle related to privacy—specifically, that people are often unaware of how their data is used. These are ethical and transparency dilemmas that cannot be overlooked, and solutions are required. Artificial intelligence (AI) has entered our lives, especially in health care, with applications and software able to autonomously set up treatment and care plans for patients. AI provides "reasoned" information to health-care professionals to best assist their work, allowing them to prescribe the best possible care.

Several companies around the world have built tools for use in AI-based health care. Deepmind Health, a company incorporated by Google Health, is one of them, and it has developed an AI program that can understand and process thousands of data and medical information in only a few minutes, to then translate it into services.

AI and its applications are experiencing a time of rapid advancement, particularly in the area of machine learning (ML). The most used machine learning, known as supervised ML, is software capable of learning to classify a set of data from the analysis of many similar cases, previously categorized by humans. The source of fuel for this process is big data, the extensive digital data sets made available, for example, by diagnostic equipment or the digitization of medical records. The machine learning approach can be applied in multiple fields, from image detection to understanding genetic data, from diagnosis through digital phenotype to drug development. Based on these factors, it is reasonable to imagine an increasing collaboration between people and artificial intelligence, where the clinical reality will become more and more data-centric, so that every detection, decision, and therapeutic intervention will be codified and recorded. It will be crucial that educational curricula of all medical professions include familiarization with these technologies, which will become increasingly important as day-to-day tools and working partners.

In addition, the use of artificial intelligence is also entering into the health-care sector. For example, in Japan, a new AI-assisted endoscopic system that would be able to identify colon and rectal adenomas during colonoscopy has recently been tested in a clinical setting. To achieve this, the diagnostic method uses an endocytoscopic image of a polyp enlarged 500 times and analyzes about 300 qualities of the polyps examined. Comparing the characteristics of each polyp with those of more than 30,000 reference images has allowed this smart probe to diagnose the presence of a dangerous lesion in less than a second with staggering precision.

Roberto's View

AI and ML have transformed the travel industry, which went from brick-and-mortar travel agencies to search engines and aggregators that can suggest the best values and prices. They've also disrupted the music business, which has moved from albums in the record store to songs in apps and digital platforms. Transforming the world of health care is something else entirely because it is a theme that touches our very humanity. Today we are the integrators of the health-care system because we go to a medical center and we generate a medical record. And once that data is collected, if we would like to reuse it, we have to request it and physically withdraw it. Thanks to new technologies, integration with the health-care system will become data driven. Instead of labs, hospitals, and doctors' offices collecting and storing data, it will be the patient who directly collects a huge amount of data and information and has it available for personal use and for analysis and mass screening. Patients will always have immediate access to their own medical records, as well as those of the health-care professional or to the health-care facilities they frequent. These records will constantly be updated to reflect a person's most current vital signs. Perhaps medical data will be made available to the scientific community for large-scale processing of predictive patterns of this or that pathology.

Technological innovation is making data analysis and its interpretation increasingly faster. One important benefit of this is greater attention to the direct relationship between the health-care professional and the patient. Big data is already everywhere, and it can be analyzed and studied for health-related issues—sometimes in unexpected ways. For example, in Switzerland, a digital epidemiologist geolocated tweets on health-related issues. In just two weeks of analysis, he was able to draw a geographical map that indicated the frequency and distribution of the messages, managing to draw useful information on the propagation of a given infection. It is a very simple use of big data from Twitter, yet it has resulted in a surprising tool, as well as one that has been extremely useful for the health-care professional. If we raise the level of analysis complexity, then it becomes clear that the impact could be more meaningful. The elaboration of these and other data could give rise to many other fundamental aspects related to the health of each one of us.

Conversa Health

Conversa, founded in 2014, with headquarters in San Francisco, California, has developed a new, simple, and effective method for patients to communicate with their health-care team. Conversa has created a library of more than 1,000 smart conversation programs on many medical issues, including asthma, chronic obstructive pulmonary disease (COPD), congestive heart failure, diabetes, hypertension, and many others, through which it can offer automated and personalized doctor–patient conversation experiences. These lead to more informed and meaningful relationships with patients, more efficient management, better clinical outcomes and, last but not least, a significant economic savings. Thanks to Conversa and to the data from more than 400 biometric devices, combined with clinical data of the patients and their feedback, the teams of health-care professionals can process the data in real time, making the distribution of health-care resources more efficient and adjusting care plans continuously, bringing them where they are needed. Coversa's digital controls use data-driven algorithms to generate clinical questions, reminders, and personalized alerts for each patient's profile. All the data received (and generated) by patients is included in the patient's electronic medical record and in the management system of his or her health assistance, which makes it possible for the teams of health-care professionals to respond quickly to the needs that may arise and to monitor people's health over time.

To date, there are several U.S. health-care facilities that use the Conversa platform to offer smart, automated conversation experiences based on patient profiles. These include, among others, Northwell Health, Ochsner Health System, Citrus Valley Health Partners, and Penrose St. Francis Health Services. The results seem to be impressive. For instance, among patients who had joint replacement surgery, there was a 20 percent reduction in care because of reduced need. This led to an average savings of $3,400 per patient over a 90-day period. More than 80 percent of the patients using Conversa's automated conversation experience said they felt more involved in their treatment.

One Drop

One Drop is an integrated system consisting of a wireless glucometer having essential and futuristic lines. It is also an app available on iOS and Android in 10 different languages, including Russian, Arabic, and Chinese. One Drop is used by people with diabetes in more than 200 countries around the world.

Thanks to One Drop, users can set up alerts for taking their medications, they can view their blood glucose data and its evolution over time, obtain statistical averages, set goals, track weight trends, see insights based on the recorded data, and provide and receive support from community users who can offer tips and advice to help them manage their diabetes. The full integration with Apple Health, Google Fit, Dexcom, and Fitbit allows One Drop users to cross-reference their blood glucose data with those related to fitness and nutrition, and to obtain other information useful for their overall health. The ability to integrate the surveys makes it possible to reduce the need for continuous attention to manual monitoring of the functions related to physical activity, duration and quality of sleep, and heart rate. To further deepen its level of knowledge, One Drop exploits the enormous potential of its database providing the community that it has gone on to build with more detailed indications. One of the most important goals for the foreseeable future, at least in the United States, is to connect health-care professionals to the One Drop information network, providing them with a more detailed picture of their patients' situations, making it possible to help them establish personalized treatments. To ensure this technology can be used by as many people as possible, One Drop offers its services and supplies for diabetes also on a monthly subscription, thus allowing people to have the daily management tools they need without the obligation of insurance, prescriptions, appointments, and so forth. Subscription plans include glucose measurement through the wireless glucometer, home delivery of glycemic test supplies, and 24/7 support from expert diabetologists. One Drop is available in the United States, Canada, the European Union, and the United Kingdom, and it can also be purchased using platforms such as Walmart, Amazon, and Best Buy, helping many people improve the way they manage diabetes.

In 2019, One Drop launched an AI-based predictive algorithm that can forecast blood-sugar levels up to eight hours out using Fitbit activity detectors and Dexcom glucose monitoring systems. In August 2020, the company signed a licensing and investment agreement worth $40 million with Bayer for the use of its technology in other sectors such as oncology, cardiology, and women's health. Starting in 2021, One Drop joined forces with Bayer and SCOR, the fourth-largest global reinsurer, to bring its AI-powered digital health platform to life for insurance carriers and policyholders across the United States.

Sensely.com

In the United States, a team of scientists is working to bring a human face to telemedicine. I am talking about Sensely, a San Francisco–based digital health and insurtech platform, which has developed a virtual nurse that can help health-care professionals and patients monitor and manage patient health in a new and efficient way. With a smiling face and a reassuring voice, the avatar designed by Sensely is a computer interface that uses ML to support the chronically ill between medical visits.

The incredibly realistic nurse avatar, amicably nicknamed Molly, was designed to have access to a patient's records so it can ask appropriate questions about the patient's past history and respond to new requests. Molly has a kind and thorough demeanor that puts the patient at ease, and interacting with the avatar is a surprisingly natural process. Molly responds to patients' requests, interacts in discussions, and is able to interpret the movements of a patient's body. When a patient needs to be "visited" by Molly, he or she poses in front of a Kinect sensor, an accessory that is movement-sensitive and was originally developed by Microsoft for the Xbox 360 gaming console. Kinect can capture a patient's image and relative position in space and send it to Molly. Once this has been done, the person states what his or her problem is. Suppose the patient is undergoing therapy for the reduction of a bursitis. He or she can raise the affected arm and show Molly, who will be able to determine if the therapy is obtaining the desired results. The Kinect sensor's skeletal tracking capabilities allow Sensely to measure the patient's range of movement and calculate changes since his or her last visit or interaction. Additionally, since the Kinect sensor records a clear view of the patient, Molly can guide him or her through appropriate therapeutic exercises. A growing number of health-care professionals and hospitals are recognizing the value of applications like Sensely. San Mateo Medical Center in California is one of several U.S. hospitals that have recently "hired" Molly to be part of their staff. The added value of such solutions is particularly evident in the treatment of patients who suffer from long-term pathological conditions and therefore require frequent monitoring of certain parameters such as blood pressure or blood sugar.

Remote treatment of a patient is less expensive and generally more efficient than on-site assistance. For this reason, solutions such as Sensely also offer a clear cost advantage to providers and insurers. A recent study has shown that Sensely reduced patient calls to health-care professionals by 28 percent, and freed nearly one-fifth of the day for those health-care professionals involved in the study. But above all, the Sensely nurse offers the promise of improved results, more frequent health monitoring and greater involvement of patients in their own care. It's something to think about the next time you're waiting in your doctor's waiting room.

The company recently closed a round of investments worth $15 million, finalized at increasing the number of languages available on the platform, to further expand into North America, Europe, the Middle East, Asia, and Australia.

SkinVision

A Dutch company has developed the SkinVision app, which is able, thanks to a photograph taken with a person's smartphone and through special algorithms, to detect some forms of skin cancer. Initially the application was focused on the detection of melanoma, but subsequent improvements and refinements of the recognition algorithm now allow the app to identify other types of cancer such as basal cell carcinoma (BCC) and squamous cell carcinoma (SCC). There are many people in the world at risk of developing skin cancer (more than one billion every year) and SkinVision can be a useful diagnostic tool, mainly thanks to the speed with which it returns results. SkinVision helps many people assess and monitor the health of their skin in all areas of the body by helping them recognize early risk indicators. This allows them to gain valuable time on diagnosis and possible treatment. The SkinVision app makes it possible for a person to create a seamless connection with his or her dermatologist to continuously monitor skin lesions, thus building a personal archive that can be referred to during visits, facilitating the work of the dermatologist and improving the quality of care.

Melanoma is a type of skin cancer that forms in the cells responsible for skin pigmentation, known as melanocytes. Although it is less common than other forms of skin cancer, it is unfortunately among the most aggressive types. There are about 132,000 cases of melanoma diagnosed each year worldwide. There are also 3 million cases of other types of skin tumors diagnosed globally. Early diagnosis allows people with melanoma to get the care they need quickly. SkinVision is able to provide concrete help for assessing the danger of an irregular spot, mole, strange pigmentation, or birthmark with an accuracy in diagnosis reaching up to 95 percent. The company has built a portfolio of 1.2 million users worldwide and a database of 3.5 million images of skin areas, both suspect and benign.

The mission of the Amsterdam-based company is to empower everyone to make the early diagnosis of skin cancer more efficient, something that is extremely important for determining treatment options. The goal of Erik de Heus, founder and CEO of SkinVision, is to save 250,000 lives over the next decade.

Guest Perspectives

JEFF DACHIS
CEO, One Drop

Jeff Dachis is one of the most well-known figures in the American tech scene. In 1994, he founded one of the first digital transformation firms, Razorfish.

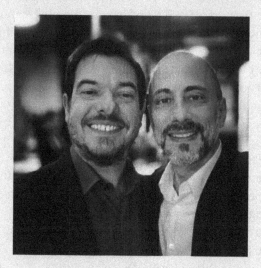

Jeff Dachis and Roberto Ascione
Credit: Roberto Ascione (Author)

In 2008, Jeff Dachis founded Dachis Group, a company that uses proprietary data analytics technology to help brands optimize their social marketing performance. In 2014, the group was acquired by Sprinklr. But the real turning point in his life came in 2013, when he turned 47 and was diagnosed with type 1 diabetes. "I remember going to the doctor and talking to the nurse for a few minutes. Then they gave me an insulin pen, a prescription, and a pat on the shoulder. I really felt neglected." Since then, he has given himself a mission: to use new technologies for improving the lives of every person with diabetes. The result was One Drop, an app whose goal is to help people with diabetes record, learn, and share information so that they can better manage the disease. But Dachis' vision goes further: "Increasingly inexpensive pervasive sensors, increasingly powerful smartphones, and giant cloud-computing environments will transform health care as we now know it. Not only will interactions between patients and health care professionals be drastically altered, but thanks to the real-time access to the patients' biometric data, the work of health-care professionals and paramedics will also be better and more efficient. Thanks to the unprecedented possibility of having real-time access to the telemetry of their biometric data, the entire procedure of delivering health care will undergo an overwhelming transformation. This huge 'evolutionary leap' will transform the role of the health care professional into something very different from how we understand it today, with a good part of the work that will be carried out by the computing power of cloud computing. This will be possible both for the volume and for the quality of the data available, combined with the ability of giving the data an intelligible meaning through the algorithms of artificial intelligence. This data can be compared with those of the medical literature, as well as with all the knowledge concerning it (especially when it will be possible to consult those anonymized cases of the various digital health records, allowing diagnosis on a global scale). Health-care techniques will be improved, the cost of care will fall dramatically, the health-care professionals and paramedics will be employed in a better and more efficient way. And all this will happen thanks to better processing of the data."

MONIQUE LEVY
Chief Commercial and Strategy Officer, WOEBOT

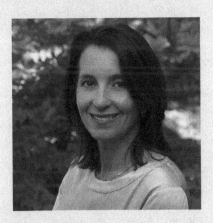

Monique Levy
Credit: Monique Levy – Private archive

Relational agents represent the most profound shift in digital health to date, and the most exciting application of AI, conversational UX, and other technologies combined.

(*Continues*)

(Continued)

Relational agents are software designed to build and maintain a social-emotional bond with users over time, and to enhance or help the user in some way, such as shifting cognition and affect to new behaviors, decisions, and knowledge. The concept of a relational agent was first discussed more than 20 years ago, most notably at MIT Media Lab's Affective Computing Group, which developed and evaluated an exercise advisor system to explore interactions between people and relational agents. The lab's study[1] found user ratings along the lines of respect, trust, and likeability were higher for the relational agent than those for the non-relational agent. A decade later another study[2] demonstrated that "individuals were more willing to disclose to an artificially intelligent 'virtual therapist' than when they believed it was human-operated."

Today's relational agents are capable of so much, but one of their more exciting applications is in the area of mental health, and one of the most innovative companies in the space is Woebot Health, where I am the chief commercial and strategy officer.

Woebot Health is the company pioneering industrializing relational agents for various unmet needs in mental health, and the first to apply them to CBT-based therapy. Its relational agent, Woebot, is accessible via apps that use a conversational UX. Woebot is built from core principles of human relationships and therapeutic process and enables people to more deeply engage with their mental health in the moment, and stay engaged as new episodes emerge over a lifetime. Woebot is also capable of quickly building a bond with users. *Bond,* or *therapeutic alliance* in clinical terms, reflects the rapport that develops between participants and Woebot. In psychotherapy, close rapport between therapist and client is a predictor of the level of change achieved. Woebot has recently demonstrated an ability to show human-level bond in a large-scale study using a standard validated measure of therapeutic relationship. Results show that Woebot can quickly create a bond non-inferior to human therapists, and maintains that bond over time, which can lead to improved mood, deeper engagement in treatment, and improved outcomes.

Woebot was created by Alison Darcy, PhD, a clinical research psychologist and health-tech visionary who believes in technology's ability to unlock human potential. Dr. Darcy built her first digital mental health solution way back in 2001. Since then, she has built an international reputation for her scientific research. At Stanford, Dr. Darcy worked with AI pioneer Andrew Ng to explore the intersection of AI and health-care, leading to his Health Innovation Lab in Computer Science. And as founder of Woebot Health, she formed the foundational ideas for an on-demand digital therapist that can support people across the lifespan. Now, Woebot is at the heart of Woebot Health's next-generation digital therapeutics for anxiety and depression, which provide the scalable innovation that can deliver trusted and effective mental health care to millions of people simultaneously.

Notes

1. Bickmore, Thomas W. and Rosalind W. Picard. "Subtle expressivity by relational agents." Available at: https://dam-prod.media. mit.edu/x/files/pdfs/03.bickmore-picard.pdf.
2. Lucas, Gale M. et al. "It's only a computer: Virtual humans increase willingness to disclose," *Computers in Human Behavior* 37, August 2014, 94–100. Available at: https://www.sciencedirect. com/science/article/abs/pii/S0747563214002647?via%3Dihub.

CHAPTER 3

Evolution of the Computer-Human Interfaces in Health Care

"The world we live in is a cacophonous environment." This curious quote is from David Rose, a researcher at the MIT Media Lab and a keen observer of how everyday life is carried out in an environment full of digital objects. The cacophony he refers to is due to the enormous number of interfaces and data by which technology has been imposing itself upon us in recent years.

Rose, an experienced designer, serial inventor, and entrepreneur, is also the author of the book *Enchanted Objects*, in which he describes a possible direction that design could take. If this were to happen, the world would be less cacophonous, populated by everyday objects made more useful and intuitive by a skillful mix of the Internet of Things (IoT), artificial intelligence (AI), and, according to Rose's personal vision of the future, "a touch of magic." The book explores how pervasive computation can become part of everyday life. Computation is the process of redistributing some of the useful things that digital technology can do for us and integrating them into the ordinary objects that already surround us. David Rose's team, for example, has developed smart pill containers, which, thanks to constant and gentle reminders in the form of light and sound, have been shown to improve the patient's ability to follow a given treatment. In fact, it is not difficult to imagine ways through which well-designed products with easy, intuitive, and beautiful interfaces will help people become better patients, help health-care professionals make the right decisions, and allow hospitals to be more efficient.

But there is a flipside to all of this, and it is that all pervasive technologies involve privacy issues. Recording a massive amount of personal information and uploading it to one's social networks or sending it through cloud-based services to have it processed poses serious problems in this regard. Not to mention the dubious ethical position of their use in marketing. Without adequate security measures and detailed privacy information, people immersed in a world like this might feel, according to David Rose's hypothesis, like the inmates of the Panopticon, the 360-degree prison designed in 1791 by Jeremy Bentham. In the Panopticon, inmates were constantly under surveillance by invisible and omniscient guards. Privacy and ethics are two issues that need to be solved and with which we will probably have to come to terms if we want to significantly improve our living and health conditions. Looking at today's world, we can already catch a glimpse of tomorrow's interfaces. One of these is virtual reality (VR), and an example of it in the health field comes from England. In a research published in the *British Journal of Psychiatry Open*, researchers at the University College of London described a new experimental therapy based on virtual reality that could help combat depression. The therapy, which involves three sessions of about 45 minutes each, was tested on 15 people suffering from depression between the ages of 23 and 61. In the first session of the experiment, participants wore a VR helmet, which allowed them to view a full-size adult avatar that replicated their movements as if they were in front of a mirror. The goal was to have the patient identify with the virtual character, so that he or she could gradually learn to be less self-critical.

In the second session, within the virtual scene there is the avatar of a child in tears, which the patient must try to console through gestures and words. In the last session, the researchers reverse the roles: the participant suddenly finds himself in the virtual body of the child and it is he or she who is comforted by the adult avatar that repeats the same words that the subject had uttered a short time earlier to console the avatar child. The trial, according to the scholars, provided "promising" results. In the month following the sessions, nine of the 15 participants reported a reduction in depressive symptoms. In particular, four experienced a "significant decline in the severity of the pathology." This is just one example of using virtual reality as a therapeutic tool, but many more are on the way.

In the near future, we will find new interfaces also in the operating room in the form of robot nurses. A study published in the journal *Frontiers in Robotics and AI* by researchers at Milan's Politecnico and Delft's University of Technology claims that androids capable of mimicking human behavior could effectively cooperate with people in high-stress situations, such as during surgeries, thus improving safety.

Immersive interfaces such as augmented reality (AR) and VR are set to play a big role in health both for patients and doctors. AR adds digital information (data, images, etc.) on top of reality, usually through connected glasses, while VR, as the name suggests, offers a fully digital virtual world to move and interact within. AR is being already successfully tested by surgeons to layer critical information (i.e., CT or MRI scans, etc.) on the view of the patients they are operating on, but we can also think of a clinical setting where the doctor is able to access lab data of the patient during the consultation, avoiding the need to focus on the computer. VR finds its application in a number of settings, including training and medical education (e.g., simulating surgical interventions), but it is also proving to be very valuable as a therapeutic intervention in many areas where a controlled and personalized stimulus is key. A good example is rehabilitation by suggesting controlled movements, or the treatment of phobias by proposing personalized scenarios that incrementally help patients to overcome their specific fears.

Roberto's View

VR, AI, robotics—there is another very interesting platform on which a feverish experimentation is taking place, based on the use of the most natural interfaces that we have: the voice and hearing. Learning how to communicate through the voice is one of the first things we do as human beings, and it's been at least since the time of *Star Trek* that we've been dreaming of turning to a computer and asking it questions, simply by calling its name.

Today, we can make an iPhone react by calling it by its name, making the 1966 dream a reality. In the field of human-computer voice interface, great strides are being made, including in the health field. There are platforms that can now be used by anyone, such as Echo, Amazon's Alexa platform, or Google Home that make it possible to create applications that we can question through voice to receive appropriate vocal responses. An interface of this type could have a huge positive impact for patients. People could ask questions about some of their symptoms and receive advice, they could set an alarm to remember when to take a pill or a specific medicine, they may get guidance about what to eat in relation to their pathology, and they could know if a certain drug should be taken with or between meals. They can, therefore, get a competent audio response without having to open an app. But the impact would also be positive on the professional front. For example, a health-care professional could get salient information about a patient during, or before, a visit, by using the smart assistant on the spot. The aspects of the interfaces are also studied from the point of view of the consumer of robotics. There is a particular trial in California that sees older people as the end-users. The robot developed by the Californian experimenters has both a voice interface and a tactile interface, thanks to which certain information can be confirmed with a touch. The very interesting thing is that, thanks to the camera with which the robot is equipped, and especially thanks to the algorithm developed by the researchers, the robot interprets the person's facial expression, understanding whether the person's expression is happy, sad, worried, and so on. Based on the data, it determines how to start a conversation whose tone is appropriate to the recognized expression. Over time, the robot not only learns how to relate to its interlocutor, but it also learns from the teachings that all other robots in the same category accumulate over time and with which it exchanges information and data. An empathetic factor that has proven to be very interesting for older people living alone.

Alexa and Echo

When Jeff Bezos beat the competition in 2014 by launching the first generation of speakers with an artificial intelligence support, it seemed almost like science fiction—and in a certain sense, it was. It was Bezos himself who confessed that the idea came to him by watching *Star Trek*, where the *Enterprise*'s on-board computer could be activated by the human voice. In fact, that's exactly what Amazon's Echo smart speakers (equipped with Alexa technology) do. Just say "Alexa" or "Amazon" aloud, and the speaker puts itself in listening mode, then records the command and responds with an action. Since 2014, thanks mainly to Amazon's agreements with major home appliance manufacturers, Alexa-based digital support has had significant growth. Thanks to Alexa's algorithms and computing ability, *domotics* (i.e., *domestic robotics*) is becoming increasingly present in homes. If, at the start, we could ask for the weather conditions before leaving the house, order a piece of music to be played, or know the appointments on our agenda, today we can ask Echo to prepare our coffee, turn on the TV or washing machine, or adjust the temperature of the boiler.

Alexa works in the same way as Siri, Cortana, and Google Assistant, the other actors in the field of speech recognition. Its strength lies in the complicated neural network developed by Amazon to decipher the commands, which allows the AI to interact with people in a simple and fluid way, and in the Echo's very sensitive microphones, which pick up the voice even if there is noise or music in the background. This type of technology has also attracted attention in the health-care field. According to Rich Able, Chief Marketing Officer of X2 Biosystems and of the Stratos Group, Alexa and Echo would be able to not only improve the inefficient health-care management systems of the United States, but they could also allow physicians and health-care personnel to have protocols of transcription and voice acquisition procedures, which would greatly improve their efficiency in the workplace.

Not only that, but by detecting changes in the intonation and character of a patient's voice Alexa's technology could also provide important clues about his or her emotional state, suggesting to the subject, where necessary and before his or her health conditions worsen, a virtual or telemedicine visit. "In our new health-care approach, it is essential to quickly understand the changes in a patient's health on a daily basis, to expand platforms of the Alexa type," said Rich Able. "And this means being able to develop, for example, new treatments for opioid addiction or for pain management."

Babylon and Healthily

Babylon Health is a British startup that has managed to raise over $600 million in funding for the design of an ingenious app that is able to mix AI with videos and consultations via messaging with health-care professionals and specialists. The use of AI helps to increase the validity of a diagnosis and, at the same time, reduces the waiting times for medical visits. The system, through speech recognition associated with AI, is able to understand what the symptoms communicated by a patient are, to then compare them with a copious database of pathologies, offering, at the end of the analysis, indications on how to intervene, what steps to take for a course of treatment, and suggesting, if the case requires so, which specialist to consult. The Babylon Health app also provides a guided route on the symptoms of a patient's malaise, so it can help the health-care professional to obtain a more accurate diagnosis in a shorter time.

If, after treatment, the health-care professional prescribes a drug, the digital prescription can be sent directly to the patient's pharmacy of choice, without the need for a written prescription, making the whole process as efficient as possible. Subsequently, the app is able to remind the patient when he or she has to take the prescribed medications for his or her treatment and to automatically activate itself from time to time to check if the conditions have been improving or not.

Babylon Health provides approximately 4,000 clinical consultations per day. Its creators say that, thanks to new investments, they will be able to reach 4.3 million users worldwide. And if, at the moment, Babylon Health plays more of a role to help specialists accurately identify the disease and the most appropriate treatment, the developers themselves don't hide the fact that they have a much more ambitious plan: treating people exclusively with AI.

Healthily (formerly Your.MD), like Babylon Health, is an application that allows anyone to consult a database of symptoms and to obtain indications on the correct behavior to adopt, whether or not to seek the advice of a health-care professional or pharmacy, or even if they should do nothing.

Healthily is a medically approved self-care app, combining responsive AI with trusted insights and tools, able to match patients' needs to the latest information from doctors and health-care specialists. This allows you to understand your health and take the next step with confidence, wherever you are. Used by millions of people all over the world, Healthily takes a pioneering approach to online clinical safety that has attracted the support of leading investors and health organizations.

Originally, Healthily was created with the intention of being able to be used as a more reliable alternative to search engines or thematic forums, even by those who do not have any medical knowledge. As Matteo Berlucchi, CEO of Healthily, said in an interview with the Italian newspaper, *Il Sole 24ore*, "In large American urban centers, the average waiting time for a medical examination is 18 days, and there are areas of the world where the density of health-care professionals is even lower than that. It's not our intention to give treatment to anyone; we want to suggest to people what they could do."

Healthily databases are powered by big data, which in turn, through mathematical models and specific analyses, returns results that represent diagnoses whose trustworthiness seeks to surpass that of health-care professionals. Once the nature of the disease has been identified (thanks to probabilistic rules), it suggests to the user which category of specialists to consult. Data science, AI, and machine learning are at the service of health and offer everyone clear and understandable answers, also because they are not written by medical personnel using medical language.

HoloLens

Microsoft first launched the mixed-reality device HoloLens in 2016; its successor, the HoloLens 2, appeared three years later. With the HoloLens, Microsoft has developed an augmented reality device that makes it possible to merge reality with virtual content and thereby facilitate all work processes, especially in the industrial sector. HoloLens is the first self-contained, holographic computer, enabling the engagement with a certain digital content and interaction with holograms in the real world.[1] With these advanced capabilities, this technology in combination with other applications is making headway in the health-care industry to help both students and health-care professionals, as it can create new and interactive ways of learning, building simulated environments for students and professionals to practice before engaging with real patients. There are many different apps and systems that are used in partnership with the HoloLens to better improve the health-care industry both in and out of operating rooms. Some of their features include helping with removing tumors, simulating ultrasounds and childbirth scenarios, analyzing all elements of the heart, helping the blind and deaf navigate in their environments, and completely dissecting the human body and all its internal systems and organs. While delivering his keynote at Virtual Med 2018 at Cedars-Sinai Medical Center, Rafael J. Grossmann Zamora, MD, a surgeon, educator, patient advocate, and health-care futurist, showcased the combination of HoloLens with an enabling app capable of further empowering Microsoft technology, by sharing all available wearable data from the patients to an expert or to the emergency department, improving the readiness and the outputs.[2]

MindMaze

MindMaze is a Swiss neuroscience company that is always look-ing for new solutions that will make the use of virtual reality more interesting. As *The Economist* reports, ever since the Indian group Hinduja invested in it by buying part of its capital, the Lausanne start-up joined the group of technology companies, which has a worth of more than $1 billion. One of MindMaze's products, not available for the consumer market, is called MASK, a tool that can improve human-machine interaction, achieved through the in-depth study of the human brain and collaboration with leading experts in the field. MASK, as can be effortlessly imagined, is similar in form to Google Daydream or to other virtual reality headsets, but it is very different in substance. In fact, it is able to read the electrical impulses of the face of the users who wear it and it can record the facial expression as precisely as possible. Once a person's facial expression has been captured, MASK can transmit it to a virtual reality avatar capable of replicating it to perfection.

MindMaze has also developed several other applications, includ-ing MindPlay, an inexpensive rehabilitation technology to help stroke and brain injury patients recover the use of their limbs. MindMotion, a neuro-rehabilitation platform, is the first MindMaze product to have been approved by the FDA. The platform provides access to 30 3D gaming activities for improving the recovery of patients with stroke-related injuries. The protocol developed takes advantage of VR gam-ing technology, helping patients engage in rehabilitative therapy and promoting their full recovery. The patient's movements are linked to those of a virtual avatar that guides him or her in the performance of several interactive exercises based on standardized principles of neural rehabilitation.

Pepper Robot

The first goal of Softbank Robotics, a robotics company founded in 2015 with headquarters in Tokyo, is to make Pepper the first human-oid robot capable of understanding the feelings, sensations, and moods of those surrounding it. It is not a robot capable of carry-ing out work or educational tasks, but simply a "family robot," with empathic abilities, able to dialogue and interact with family members, accompanying them pleasantly throughout their lives.

The task is not easy, but Softbank Robotics is convinced that this is a challenge it can win. After the first successes obtained in Japan, in 2017 Pepper was also launched on the U.S. market and in some European countries, and soon it will be launched in Italy. But it is Pepper's empathetic abilities that have attracted the attention of the health field. For example, in Belgium, in the AZ Damiaan hospital, Pepper is already being used to welcome patients during the acceptance procedures. Pepper looks like a small humanoid, measuring just one meter and 20 centimeters tall, and it is perfectly suited to the welcoming role since it can speak 19 languages perfectly, making it able to address virtually all incoming patients. For now, it is being tested in the maternity ward, where the feedback has been decidedly positive, especially from the younger guests. But everything about it suggests wider use and application in other departments. The era of robotic welcoming has begun!

Psious

Available in 27 countries, Psious is the first VR platform for therapists and health-care professionals working in the mental health field. Several pathologies are treated in more than 70 gaming environments, which makes it possible to experience pathological situations through VR, with constant monitoring by the therapist.

Psious offers new digital therapeutics that could be used more frequently and more quickly than traditional ones, with the objective that no one should be limited by the state of their mental health. In this way, their goal is to help people face their problems and live a full life, a life without stress, a life without anxiety, fears, or phobias.

The company has two main objectives. The first is to continue to have an increase in the number of patients they help and the number of therapists who use their product. The second is to work on the clinical side of the product, increasing the level of evidence behind their system, together with their partners, so that it becomes the most advanced and validated VR solution on the market.

"We want to achieve something meaningful: improving mental health globally," says Xavier Palomer, Psious CEO.

PatchAi

PatchAi is a startup that has developed the first cognitive platform for collection and predictive analysis in a conversational form (Co-PRO) of patient-reported data in clinical trials. They have developed an empathetic virtual assistant that constantly collects valuable data while improving the entire patient experience during clinical trials.

The idea, conceived in Italy among the hospital wards, manages to offer a personalized medical experience that puts the patient at the center, thanks to the implementation of technologies such as AI and ML.

PatchAi, with its virtual assistant, is able to interpret the needs of patients and do real-time monitoring of the engagement, adherence to the treatment, symptoms, quality of life, and other information reported by patients.

Notes

1. Limonte, Kelly. "AI in healthcare: HoloLens in surgery," Microsoft Cloudblogs, December 20, 2018. Available at: https://cloudblogs.microsoft.com/industry-blog/en-gb/health/2018/12/20/ai-healthcare-hololens-surgery/.
2. Grossman, Rafael. Talk to introduce Nomadeec HoloLens, Virtual Med 2018. Available at: https://www.youtube.com/watch?v=ocWE8nEfZ6I.

CHAPTER 4

Telemedicine and Remote Monitoring

How Telemedicine Will Change Our Lives

The term *telemedicine* was coined in the 1970s and refers to the use of information and communication technologies for improving the conditions of the patients, increasing access to treatment and to medical information.

Although there is no single definition, in 2007 the World Health Organization defined telemedicine as "the delivery of health care services, where distance is a critical factor, by all health care professionals using information and communication technologies for the exchange of valid information for diagnosis, treatment and prevention of disease and injuries..."

In the digital era, telemedicine and tele-assistance are procedures that can bring direct benefits to the patient, with clear decreases in both travel costs and social spending, also contributing to the achievement of universal health coverage.

The use of telemedicine services has opened new possibilities in the management of care pathways in developing countries, in those areas where access to care is more difficult or in situations of health emergency, such as the one caused by the Covid-19 pandemic.

It was the sudden need to address the Covid-19 pandemic that gave an unprecedented boost to the various telemedicine services in clinical practice, which in many cases have become a central asset to primary care consultations. It is no coincidence that when we talk about this massive acceleration in the use of telemedicine solutions, we can define it as a "viral uptake." In the United States, for example, between March and April 2020, one of the most critical moments of the pandemic, the multisite Mayo Clinic saw a 10,880 percent increase in video appointments. Typically, Mayo Clinic sees 1.2 million patients annually, making it the largest U.S. health-care system. Prior to the pandemic, 300 of their providers had made at least one video telemedicine visit in the previous year. By mid-July, that number had risen 2,000 percent to more than 6,500.[1]

In Europe telemedicine is reaching a maturity stage, as noted by the HIMSS e-Health Trendbarometer study conducted just prior to the Covid-19 crisis. According to the study, 93 percent of health-care facilities had implemented at least one type of telehealth service or solution, particularly those for chronic disease management. The scenario completely changed with the onset of the pandemic, demonstrating the tremendous value of telehealth in building resilient health-care systems that can adapt to new challenges.

There are still some important barriers that have to be broken down for telehealth to maximize its expansion, such as the lack of a reimbursement policy of the expenditure and how to act in the case of litigation for medical liability. Both of these issues are under discussion, but in any case, the performance of telemedicine simply requires necessary rules that translate into standard operating procedures. Telemedicine is an example of how digital technology facilitates dialogue, the sharing of different skills and knowledge, as well as easy access to data. It is precisely these three elements that will be central to any innovation process in the near future.

Patients will update the health-care professionals about their health via video, they will be able to ask questions and inquire about their health condition, and the health-care professionals will provide answers and educational content to improve adherence to the proposed treatment or to raise awareness of a particular pathology. In America, we already have a taste of the future, where the number of virtual visits (made by phone, email, or video) is greater than the number of traditional visits. The global market is expected to reach the value of $185.66 billion by 2026.

Virtual care has been catalyzing most of 2020 funding. Telemedicine, whose potential had been discussed for years, became a necessity once Covid-19 struck.

As shared by StartUp Health in their dedicated reports, telemedicine funding in Q1 2020 has been up by 1,818 percent and remote patient monitoring platforms by 168 percent.[2]

On-demand health-care services (telemedicine services, prescription delivery, and at-home urgent care) is the top-funded value proposition with $2.0 billion invested across 48 deals through Q3 2020. It is also the value proposition with the greatest number of deals. By one estimate, telemedicine claims in the United States rose by over 4,000 percent between June 2019 and June 2020.[3]

Covid-19: The Tipping Point of Telehealth

The Covid-19 global pandemic outbreak constituted a tipping point for telehealth adoption globally. As in the past, the need for an innovation fostered its adoption at scale. These solutions provided a safe tool to manage positive patients and also the many others likely infected but not tested, which are estimated to be between 1 in 5 and 1 in 10 and who need to stay home while still being monitored and assisted as needed.

These were extremely significant numbers proving strong adoption in a crisis time.

Roberto's View

Telemedicine has origins that are relatively distant, especially if one thinks in terms of digital evolution. Today, we already have devices and technologies that allow complete monitoring as well as remote monitoring of many vital parameters, although, due to costs of both production and management that are still too high, their diffusion is not yet widespread. To date, devices of this type are still all too often confined to monitoring certain particularly serious diseases, or for the use and consumption of those who can afford them. But soon the horizon is destined to be widened: the reduction of production costs and the increased ease of implementation will make it possible to create devices for a wider range of pathologies, and the spread of these devices will expand, as happened in recent years for smartphones, to ever more varied consumer groups.

The Covid-19 pandemic has accelerated the democratization of telemedicine and in particular the adoption of remote monitoring, with enormous consequences in the near future of medicine.

Thanks to telemedicine services, physicians can guarantee continuity of care and access to patients daily, even if they are dozens of kilometers away from the health-care facility, allowing them to intervene promptly and with great effectiveness. In addition, remote monitoring will allow surgeons to operate through robotic interfaces across great distances, thus combining the micrometric precision of a robot with the care and experience of the great primary surgeon—and at significantly lower management costs than are possible in the current situation. Not to mention how, thanks to this type of remote surgical operation, the participation of health-care professionals will increase, who will be able to assist, in telepresence, the operating stages in an unequalled process of learning and updating.

Omada Health

Omada Health was founded in 2011 by Sean Duffy, after he earned a master's degree in health care and medicine from Harvard in 2010. He had previous work experiences at Google and Ideo soon after he graduated in neuroscience from Columbia University in New York in 2006. This enriching background led him to believe that behavioral medicine is at an incredible turning point of innovation, thanks to technology and design, and Omada clearly embodies Sean's belief, being conceived as a digital care program that empowers patients to achieve their health goals through sustainable lifestyle change. Combining data-powered human coaching, connected devices, and curriculum tailored to patients' specific circumstances, the program is designed to help them build healthy patterns for life. In the 21st century, one in three Americans is likely to die prematurely from a condition that is closely related to lifestyle. Thus, it is vital to change habits to improve health and consequently minimize the risks of chronic diseases. At Omada, behavioral science leverages the implementation of the right tools, the right language, and the motivational ability to support people embracing a different lifestyle. Verified clinical studies have shown that, on average, in 12 months, the participants in the Omada programs see the possibility of the onset of Type 2 diabetes decrease by 30 percent, the risk of heart attack by 16 percent, and the risk of heart disease by 13 percent. In addition, already after 16 weeks, participants have recorded an average weight loss of 4 to 5 percent and, looking at the data available, this weight reduction has been maintained over time. Furthermore, Omada's estimations show that a company (which has chosen their program for their employees' health) might need two years to get its investment amortized and five years to have a net profit.

Sano

Sano is a smart patch with microinvasive technology that can measure interstitial fluid in the outer layer of the skin by continuously calculating a patient's blood sugar and sending data to an app in real time. The surface of the patch is slightly rough to the touch, similar to very light sandpaper. The texture comes from the microtubules present in the inner side of the patch that then gently penetrate into the epidermal layer, allowing the analysis of the intercellular fluids, from which the level of sugar in the metabolism is then calculated. The readings, processed by a sophisticated chip inserted into the patch, are then transmitted via Bluetooth to the app and from here are synchronized to a cloud server. Sano's technology is able to generate, in an absolutely comfortable way compared to a normal glucometer, a continuous series of data, even more than 100 per day, providing real-time blood glucose values and thus helping people to make faster and more precise decisions about their nutrition. Ashwin Pushpala, founder and CEO of Sano, said he wanted to expand the use of the technology to people who are not directly affected by diabetes. It will be useful in cases when a patient's blood sugar levels provide important information for taking preventive action or for improving one's own eating lifestyle, with a particular focus on those who are overweight or have a tendency toward obesity. In this sense, Pushpala itself does not rule out extending the use of Sano to people who want to undertake a particular diet, or even to the world of fitness. An effect related to the collection of all this big data could be the mass study at the physiological, epidemiological, and social level of the phenomenon of diabetes, to the benefit of clinical research that could have an enormous amount of data available at low cost that it can then analyze.

Teladoc Health

Teladoc Health is the leading telemedicine company in the United States. It was founded in 2002 in Dallas by Byron Brooks, a former NASA physician, and Michael Gorton, an entrepreneur. Teladoc was launched nationally in 2005 at the Consumer Directed Health Care

Conference in Chicago, Illinois. In 2007, just two years after its official launch, Teladoc had already reached nearly one million people with its services, including through some large companies that had begun to adopt the company' services as part of the health benefits for their employees. Since 2015, Teladoc has become the only telemedicine company to be listed on the New York Stock Exchange, and in December 2016, the American Hospital Association entered into an exclusive agreement to use its telematics platform. Teladoc provides registered users with access to consulting services with certified health-care professionals, 24 hours a day, for any type of standard (i.e., non-emergency) problem such as allergy, flu, conjunctivitis, and otitis through exclusive audio-video technology.

Teladoc Health is successfully transforming the way people access and experience health care, with a focus on high quality, lower costs, and improved results around the world. Ranked first among the direct-to-consumer tele-assistance service providers in the J.D. Power 2019 U.S. Telehealth Satisfaction Study, Teladoc Health's integrated services include remote assistance, expert health-care professional services, AI and analytics, and licensed platform services. With more than 2,400 employees, the organization provides health-care assistance in 130 countries and in more than 30 languages, and it collaborates with employers, hospitals, health-care systems and insurers, to transform the delivery of the treatments. In October 2020, Teladoc Health announced the completion of its merger with Livongo, a milestone marking one of the most significant blendings of capabilities in the history of digital health.

TytoCare

TytoCare is an Israeli startup that has raised $11 million for the development and marketing of a new and revolutionary medical device: a small instrument, Tyto, that makes it possible for a person to listen to the body and to obtain, immediately after, the advice of a health-care professional through a mobile platform. What makes the device unique is the fact that the algorithms associated with TytoApp (a smartphone application) and the visual recognition technologies guide users even through complicated exams. Tyto offers a comprehensive solution that allows the health-care professional to interact with the patient both online and offline, storing the patient's data and using it to improve his or her health-care assistance. In 2021, the telehealth company is continuing to expand its platform with the launch of a pulse oximeter to enable people to check their blood oxygen saturation (SpO_2) levels and heart rate at home.

VitalConnect

VitalConnect, with headquarters in the heart of Silicon Valley, was founded in 2011 with the vision of changing the health-care paradigm by creating a new world of information based on predictive data analytics. To achieve this, it created a small but very powerful device, the VitalPatch, a patch with an integrated wireless biosensor that can monitor eight critical vital signs simultaneously: heart rhythm, respiratory rate, body temperature, blood pressure, steps, body tilt (to detect loss of balance), stress level, and the stages and quality of sleep (hypnogram). The VitalPatch is particularly suitable for the elderly and makes it possible to remotely control patients with various pathologies. It can be used to obtain an immediate report on the health of a patient, from hospitals, emergency rooms, and from the trusted health-care professional. It collects thousands of data items every minute through the SensorFusion algorithm and it creates very accurate statistics. The data, encrypted according to HIPAA rules, is continuously transmitted to a cloud server that can, if necessary, send notifications by email or through the most commonly used instant messaging systems, alerting health-care professionals and family members in case of need. The solution developed by VitalConnect provides health-care professionals and the hospital staff with a continuous flow of data that health-care professionals can monitor to safeguard the patient's health or to predict events before they occur. This type of analysis can help improve the assistance for at-risk patients, for example, those with heart failure or serious infections. But it can also help predictively detect any changes in the patients' physiology, potentially decreasing mortality rates or the number of days spent in intensive care.

Guest Perspective

CARLOS NUENO
President, International Operations, Teladoc Health

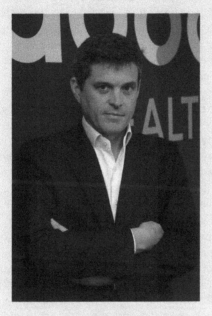

Carlos Nueno

Credit: Carlos Nueno – Private archive

Writing this paragraph in March 2021 allows me to have some perspective on the consequences of the worst global pandemic we have suffered since the early 20th century. Now that we have been more than one year battling the consequences of the coronavirus, if there is one thing that has allowed our society to continue with a certain degree of activity, it our capacity to connect with others. The wide coverage of internet, the penetration of cellular phones, the wide spread of WiFi, and in general the excellent networks of telecommunications that we have today have allowed us to transform the way we live our lives.

(Continues)

(*Continued*)

As a side effect of the pandemic, the adoption of virtual care has experienced an acceleration and has become a fundamental part of the health-care system. From physicians, to patients, to organizations and governments, all now consider virtual care as a fundamental part of their roadmap. We are already seeing how governments are incentivizing health-care systems to transform their health-care delivery, incorporating telemedicine and even starting to reimburse for digital therapies. However, what will deliver a greater value to our society is the way virtual care will be integrated into our homes, our work, our daily life and into the health-care system in general.

This transformation won't be at the expense of physicians; on the contrary it will require more professionals and more skilled ones. Physicians will be empowered by the extended capabilities provided by the integration of virtual care and technology. For example, in the United Kingdom we are already connecting GPs (primary care doctors) to consultants through technology to empower them in a matter of minutes to be able to provide a higher level of care at primary care centers. The consequence of which is an increase of resolution at the primary care level with a decrease on waiting times and costs.

In the next 5 to 10 years, we are going to see a revolution in the area of connected devices that will allow us not only to keep track of our health but also to prevent disease and connect us to the right level of care at the right point in time. At Teladoc Health, our connected devices already allow us to manage more than 1 billion data points from chronic patients. Data that our algorithms transform into actionable information allowing patients to have full control of their disease while allowing us to connect them virtually to the right health-care professional anytime, anywhere.

At Teladoc Health, we believe that in order to improve patients' lives, we must combine the capacity of connecting patients to the health-care system anytime and anywhere through virtual care, using the most advanced and secure technology, and also being able to connect patients with devices in order to monitor their health at home and prevent disease. The combination and integration of these three elements is at the core of our strategy to provide better and more sustainable care to everyone around the world.

Notes

1. Marin, Allison. "Telemedicine takes center stage in COVID-19," *Science*, November 6, 2020. Available at: https://www.sciencemag.org/features/2020/11/telemedicine-takes-center-stage-era-covid-19.
2. StartUp Health. "Health innovation sees funding boom in the lead up to COVID-19," HealthTransformer.co, April 7, 2020. Available at: https://healthtransformer.co/health-innovation-sees-funding-boom-in-the-lead-up-to-covid-19-1d19069984aa.
3. Wang, Elaine, and Sean Day. "Q3 2020: A new annual record for digital health (already)," Rock Health, n.d. Available at: https://rockhealth.com/reports/q3-2020-digital-health-funding-already-sets-a-new-annual-record/.

CHAPTER 5

Digital Health Enabling Platforms

Platforms for Connecting Doctors and Patients, Remote Monitoring Systems, and Management of Their Therapies

More than half a million health apps circulate in the various digital stores. These are variations on a theme, from those that track eating habits to those that can function as an intelligent alarm for taking drugs, from those useful for monitoring one's lifestyle to those created for making appointments for exams or specialist visits, up to those more specifically linked to the world of wellness and to support the most diversified sports activities. The digital phenomenon takes on even greater proportions when one considers the digital services and tools of interaction of health facilities and individual doctors with their patients. For example, through social networks such as Facebook or Twitter, digital tools can launch campaigns for prevention, health education, and the promotion of a healthy lifestyle. This referral to digital technology by users is an indication of their expectations for the health care of the future; that is, it evolves toward systems that are easier, more efficient, more accessible, and closer to the person. It is easy to imagine that real service platforms will emerge where it is possible for people to consult their clinical history, make appointments for diagnostic tests or specialist visits, pay for services perhaps through their own insurance, view their appointments and modify them independently, check the vaccinations carried out, receive remote consultations, and much more.

In the same way, more and more platforms are available for doctors who offer a multitude of services for the virtual management of their clinic and effectively respond to the needs of their patients.

In the not-too-distant future, therefore, we can say that each of us will have access to an integrated service platform for autonomously and safely managing every aspect of our health.

The proliferation of health platforms can be explained both as a response to assistance that becomes increasingly patient-centered as well as being linked to the growing number of channels used and their data flow. This would explain the need for hospitals or care teams to have some sort of unified dashboard, to have the entire patient's health history stored in just one place.

In the next few years we might be seeing a shift in the places where health care is provided, since the place of care will move from the hospital or clinic to anywhere the patients are—at work, at home, or wherever they are able to bring their smartphones. We therefore understand that the new generation of digital health platforms will be based on a more personalized approach to medicine, with greater attention given to primary and preventive medicine in order to also reduce access to emergency rooms and the related costs of care. An example for better understanding this topic is Piedmont Healthcare,[1] a health-care system that serves more than 2 million people in Georgia, which has decided to develop with Salesforce a single platform for having a shared view of patients with data on their medical history, insurance, scheduled appointments, and preferences. The ultimate goal is being able to provide a more coordinated and patient-oriented experience at a lower total cost of care.

With the advent of the Covid-19 pandemic, many health organizations have had to implement new communication tools, such as chatbots or telemedicine solutions, to be able to handle the sudden increase in requests from patients and/or doctors.

Italy was one of the first countries in the world, after China, to be hit hard by the Covid-19 pandemic and therefore one of the first countries where the digital health startups began to mobilize to provide solutions to the new problems that were presenting themselves. One of these, Paginemediche.it, the most widespread digital health platform in Italy, was among the first companies in the sector to respond promptly, making widely tested digital tools available to doctors and patients. It's tools could contribute to the effective management of the Covid-19 health emergency. In fact, in the space of a few weeks, Paginemediche.it adapted its telemedicine tools in order to respond to the emergency, developing three different services that were easy to access and interconnected: 1) a chatbot for the triage of the symptoms, 2) the video visit for remote consultations, and 3) home remote monitoring of Covid-19 patients.

Since February 2020, an automatic chatbot has been active on Paginemediche.it. It is clinically validated by a team of doctors and scientists and can carry out an evaluation of the symptoms of coronavirus infection in real time, suggesting the most suitable diagnostic path. This has made it a valid instrument at the institutional level, so much so that it was also made available on the websites of the Regions of Lombardy, Trentino-Alto Adige, and Campania.

The number of triages carried out in only the first months of operation has been enormous: 117,000, of which 60,000 have been brought to term.

To prevent the spread of the virus, Paginemediche.it has also developed a video visit module, made available free of charge to all Italian doctors, to carry out remote consultations in complete safety. The service was also complemented by an at-home management service of confirmed or suspected cases of Covid-19, with low and/or medium severity symptoms. Interestingly, the access to the service can take place either at the invitation of the doctor or upon the request of the patient. This created a so-called network effect which allowed the system to scale very rapidly, with relevant best practices being expanded to other diseases and conditions. As we finalize this book a scientific study has been completed and accepted for scientific publication in the *Journal of Medical Internet Research* (JMIR), demonstrating the viability of this approach.

Roberto's Vision

Let us think for a moment about the waiting lists for making appointments for medical services, whether they are for specialist or diagnostic visits. We should take the example of low-cost airlines, which are the quintessence of organizing the occupation of the places available. And yet, unfortunately, what all too often happens is that we are still inundated with waiting lists. We need to call several facilities to know if there is a spot available; we sit through long and exhausting waits on the phone, only on certain days and at certain times, and hope that luck is on our side.

The truth is that compared to platforms in other industries, health care is both more complex and more fragmented.

If it's really easy to book a flight today, it's not quite as easy to do the same for a medical consultation. If you enter "doctor online" on Google, you get more than four million results in less than a second.

Technology, even today, could meet us halfway. In fact, all it takes is the creation of a unique bot for people to communicate the type of problem (e.g., I need an eye examination, a CT scan, an MRI, an orthopedic specialist, etc.) and from which to receive fast and geolocated answers, at any time of the day and night, without too many bureaucratic delays and with less technological hurdles.

It is a huge gap to fill, but we are already seeing some important steps forward. The new normality generated by the Covid-19 pandemic has seen the emergence of new needs and new ways of interacting between doctors and patients. This is pushing for the increased use of digital tools not only for making appointments, but also for utilizing diagnostic tools, prescribing therapies and treatments, and for managing the follow-up visits.

Paginemediche's experience in Italy makes it clear that the new normal will be characterized by the use of platforms intended as actual integrated hubs that allow, in a single digital space, tools and services that best respond to the needs of the patients and doctors themselves.

In any case, the new health-care platforms open up opportunities for improving outcomes, lowering costs, and building experiences that are truly focused on the users' needs. The start of the race to the platforms can be identified in the Teladoc-Livongo agreement, the largest digital health acquisition to date, worth $18.5 billion, although there have been other players in the field for some time and in continuous evolution.

The market for digital health platforms is still highly fragmented with the presence of different platforms according to the type of services offered: from those that offer treatments for a specific group of pathologies to omnichannel ones with the possibility of purchasing drugs, diagnostic tests or remote monitoring services, up to platforms that integrate telemedicine platforms with in-person services in health-care facilities.

The question is not whether, but when platforms will assume dominance in health-care assistance, managing to play a key role in the supply, delivery, and organizing of health services thanks to a strong technological infrastructure, high customer experience, and clinical expertise.

Altibbi

Altibbi is the Middle East's largest digital health platform, operating in 10 markets across the Arab world by offering telemedicine consultation services, allowing patients to connect directly with doctors via audio calls and chats. Arabic speaking users get access to trusted and reliable health answers from a network of doctors in all specialties.

Altibbi users can subscribe to a monthly fee for an unlimited live consult with doctors with its Call Doctor service via HD voice on Android and iPhone.

Apple Health

The launch of Apple Health in 2014 coincided with version 8 of the operating system developed in Cupertino. The initial purpose of the app was to collect, with the user's consent, a series of health information within a single container, a sort of medical record of the user, using both the characteristics integrated into the various Apple devices, and the incoming data from the various trackers that were beginning to have a considerable distribution on the consumer market. Over the years, Apple Health has been enhanced with new features and today the goal of Apple's medical technology team is to transform the app from a simple data collection tool to a diagnostic tool. The biggest stumbling block to overcome is that of creating a common standard of display of the collected data, so that it can be read from different databases. If this data could be interpreted by data processing tools from different health-care facilities, the work of doctors would be greatly facilitated, allowing them to obtain funda-mental information coming from a huge amount of data.

In the words of Apple CEO Tim Cook, "Health is a matter of great importance around the world and we think it's time to simplify some aspects of it and propose new points of view." Not forgetting that, in addition to this laudable aspect, the operation is also of great value in terms of economic return. To achieve its goal in early 2017, Apple purchased Gliimpse, a startup that specializes in creating tools that make it possible for one to manage and share his or her own per-sonal medical data.

A few weeks after the acquisition, it was Mohan Randhava, the senior engineer in charge of Apple Health (as well as former Gliimpse engineer) who wrote on his LinkedIn profile that he was "working on building a platform, a series of APIs (application program inter-faces) and a simple product that allows us to obtain what we believe is an explosive application in the field of health care." Since 2015, Apple has in fact made ResearchKit available, an open-source plat-form to develop apps that make it much easier to conduct scientific studies and find patients willing to participate in them. The effect was, as Randhava predicted, explosive. Using ResearchKit to conduct studies allowed researchers to target a larger and more diverse group of participants, as well as making it possible to collect a continuous flow of data from sensors and devices, such as had never been possible before. This new way of collecting data has led to interesting discoveries in the field of sound engineering, active vision, women's health, and cardiology.

As may be readily self-evident, Apple is transforming HealthKit into a useful tool for making diagnoses. It will be easy to consult not only for users, but also for doctors and hospitals, thanks to the use of the Apple Watch and iPhone and in collaboration with academic medical institutions and research communities.

Cohealo

Cohealo is an American technological company that has developed an effective system for connecting the hospitals scattered throughout the United States so that facilities that need specific medical-diagnostic equipment can request it (for rent) from other health-care units that are not using it at that time. Cohealo's goal is, therefore, to optimize the use of technological equipment and infrastructure, typically a very expensive process. To help various hospital facilities across different departments, Cohealo uses the same idea that Airbnb had for facilitating rental of rooms and houses to tourists. In the case of Airbnb, private individuals do not intend to use the rental properties for a given time of year. To optimize hospital technology among different departments, Cohealo can help clarify when different tools and equipment are planned to be in use.

The creation of Cohealo is due to Mark Slaughter, the company's current CEO, formerly a dealer of electronic equipment for operating rooms. Thanks to his profession in sales, as early as 2010, Slaughter was aware of some hidden problems in the American health-care system, but the real intuition that allowed him to invent Cohealo had come to him through thorough study of the numerical data. Slaughter noticed a significant fact: over the course of a year, in many hospitals the equipment remained unused for as much as 75 percent of the time. Bingo! Slaughter's idea was to build a centralized system of information on the instruments used in the health-care facilities in order to allow the various departments to monitor the rates of use of the devices, allowing them to be able to promptly move them according to the various needs. Alternatively, it allows clinics to be mapped according to the specialization of the diagnostic and medical machines, so that patients who need specific treatments can effectively be addressed to these facilities, thus increasing the rates of use of the devices. Using Cohealo reduces the need for health-care facilities to buy machines that won't be fully utilized. This brings about an obvious economic advantage. It's easy to be a prophet if you assume that in the near future, to optimize resources and reduce costs, platforms like Cohealo will be increasingly used.

DocDoc

DocDoc is a Singapore-based health-tech startup that uses technology in conjunction with medically trained professionals to optimize health-care outcomes and cost and enhance the patient's end-to-end health-care journey. The company combines AI-powered doctor discovery, telemedicine, and digital third-party administrator services onto a single platform. With this platform, DocDoc enables insurance companies, brokers, employers, and governments to reduce health-care costs, improve the frequency and quality of engagement as well as allow them to offer a customized health-care experience. The startup operates in eight countries with more than 23,000 doctors in its network.

Doctolib

Turning to "Dr. Google" when the first symptoms of a disease arise is a well-known phenomenon, but the user is not only looking for immediate solutions to his or her malaise or information that can explain the cause (however right or wrong these personal interpretations may be). Often, if necessary, one also looks for a specialist to contact for a consultation or visit. For some years now, technological and digital solutions that allow one to make appointments for visits and specialist examinations are gaining ground around the world. The French Doctolib is one of them.

Founded in 2013, it accelerated rapidly, first at home and then in other countries of the European community, until opening another office in Berlin in 2018.

Currently, there are about 30 million monthly appointments that pass through Doctolib, a remarkable number that has beneficial consequences for patients as well as for doctors. It even offers advantages for the entire national health system, which Doctolib manages, to direct patients much more efficiently than in the past. The scope of Doctolib's business is potentially huge. Every month there are about 25 million appointments with the presence on the platform of 65,000 doctors and professionals, operating in 1,300 health facilities.

hi.health

The services offered by hi.health were launched in Germany at the end of 2019. Within a few months, it had been used by thousands of people for managing reimbursements (almost half a million euros) to their private insurance companies.

hi.health aims at making medical service packages accessible and customizable on a large scale. The company achieves this by integrating innovations from the fintech sector into health insurance, allowing the direct payment and billing of health-care expenses.

This, combined with a strong focus on personal service, powers the team concierge, which creates a more direct and personal way of managing what was once a routine task. By interfacing with providers of digital health-care products, online consulting, pharmacies, and logistics companies, hi.health informs users directly, and provides access to such offers—without problems—dealing with the management of requests, payments, and reimbursements.

Livongo

Founded in 2014, Livongo offers diverse digital services and products to support people in the management of chronic diseases such as diabetes or high blood pressure.

According to Livongo, chronic diseases can be managed more effectively and can be more economically sustainable through an offer that integrates software, wearables, and personalized coaching programs. In this way, the more than 164,000 members of the services developed by Livongo are able not only to collect aggregated data on their health conditions, but also to share this data with their doctors, who can interpret it in real time. In August 2020, Livongo merged with Teladoc, the global leader in whole-person virtual care, with the aim of creating a new type of health experience, which allows people to live in a healthier way. The two companies together managed to deliver about 10.6 million virtual visits in 2020.

Paginemediche

Paginemediche.it is the Italian digital health platform that connects doctors and patients and offers a personalized health experience. It was founded in 2001 as a web portal on health and medicine, soon becoming a market leader and increasing its notoriety in only a few short years. In 2016 it was renewed by integrating content and services with high added value for patients, consumers, and health professionals into a single solution. Today it is an integrated platform, able to offer personalized health programs and to respond to the most diverse needs that intervene in the relationship between doctors and patients as the main players of the digital change that we are experiencing in the health sector, from making appointments for visits to the possibility of taking advantage of teleconsulting and video consultation. On Paginemediche, the users have access to a dedicated dashboard for the control and management of their own health, with personalized contents and services based on individual biometric parameters and preferences. Doctors have at their disposal a management system for the organization and development of their professional activities. They can access various services to support optimized patient management, from the ability to make appointments 24/7 to booking management, from telemedicine to patient management, providing for a comprehensive tool to digitalize the patient journey.

In 2020, more than 20 million users accessed Paginemediche and took advantage of the platform's services, which include more than 11,000 professionals active in telemedicine.

Paginemediche represents a true hub of digital health, able to bring doctors and patients together and provide simple but rigorous solutions to the many users who turn to it.

This ability has led Paginemediche to make its services available on Italy's days of maximum alert for coronavirus. Specifically, a chatbot has been developed using guidelines of the Italian Ministry of Health to support doctors during triage and avoid the overload of ordinary telephone lines, greatly speeding up the process of identifying persons who may be infected with the novel coronavirus and, at the same time, giving the user the opportunity to access a full at-home management of Covid-19 patients which had a huge positive impact during the pandemic. Frost & Sullivan has nominated Paginemediche as one of the ten "Digital Technologies Helping Humans in the Fight Against COVID-19."[2]

Guest Perspectives

MARC SLUJIS
Managing Partner, DigitalHealth.Network

Marc's passionate about scaling the digital health sector as facilitator of M&A, growth investment, and strategic partnerships.

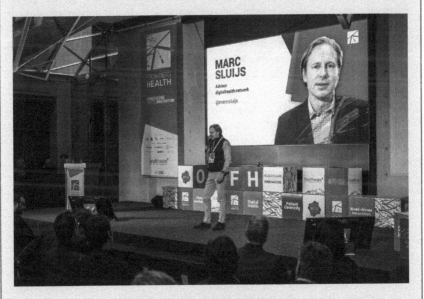

Marc Slujis at Frontiers Health
Credit: Frontiers Health

(*Continues*)

(Continued)

For the past six years, Marc has been advising large investors (EQT, Mubadala) as well as life sciences companies with regard to mergers and acquisitions (M&A), fundraising, and investment in digital health and digital therapeutics. He is an advisor to several digital therapeutics companies and is also helping digital health companies achieve scale and exit. Marc shares:

Having been exclusively focused on digital health for 11 years, including M&A and investment, Marc has identified several things that seem very obvious. There is a tremendous amount of innovation in digital health, which is fabulous. At the same time, however, the vast majority of companies in this sector are subscale, and will therefore not make any meaningful impact on the world. It's the lack of scale that's the biggest obstacle to adoption, and not whether there are reimbursement codes or not.

The lack of scale manifests itself in three major hurdles:

1. Most digital health companies only provide a piece of the broader solution, which makes adoption extremely complex, and hence barely feasible. It's unrealistic to expect from large health-care providers, payers, or pharma companies that they will be able to: (a) select the different components of a complete solution, (b) understand how these should all fit together, and (c) operationalize this complex construct. The "point solution challenge" is further exacerbated by the fact that many founders lack the realization that they only represent a small piece of a bigger puzzle and lack a good understanding of how their small piece could/should fit in the bigger scheme of things.
2. There is a lack of bandwidth to deliver solutions internationally. This makes it difficult to partner with multinational clients who seek to have a single supplier for their programs.
3. The lack of financial stability of many digital health companies means they often cannot be considered as viable partners by large organizations. It is not realistic to expect large organizations to embark on strategic programs that impact their patients, physicians, payers, and other stakeholders with subscale companies with limited financial runway due to the high level of inherent risk.

In order to mitigate these challenges, there's an urgent need for:

- An acceleration of M&A to bring the pieces of the puzzle together and create scale quicker—this will require entrepreneurs to think more proactively about M&A, and to ensure that they build their solution and company to facilitate integrations. Also, this requires investors to be more supportive of early stage nonorganic growth strategies and provide (more) funding accordingly.

- More concentrated investment in the right assets (that also have management teams with the skillsets to build, integrate and lead bigger entities). In addition to growth VC investment, there is a marked opportunity for earlier stage buy and build fund strategies.
- Meaningful partnerships beyond the pilots that many have been playing around with for too long and that offer consumers a disproportionate amount of resources from startups, and have too little strategic or financial impact.

Fortunately, there are several positive indicators, the most important probably being the strong growth in interest of large investors. Through my regular contacts with hundreds of investors ranging from growth venture capitalists, family offices, and private equity to sovereign wealth funds, collectively managing more than $3 trillion, it is evident that there is a big appetite to invest more in health-care technology and digital health. The key challenge currently is that there is a lack of assets that have enough scale for these investors to deploy the amount of capital available. However, as we are nearing a tipping point, the next five years will be seeing a massive inflow of investment from larger funds, which should enable the digital health sector to scale to its full potential.

ALI HASAN
Chief Medical and Healthcare Officer, Vitality

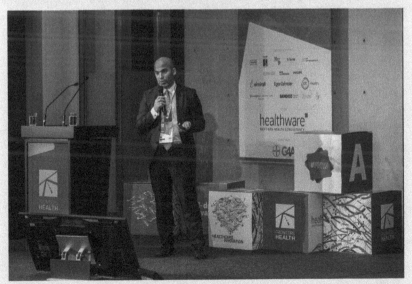

Ali Hasan at Frontiers Health
Credit: Frontiers Health

(*Continues*)

(Continued)

The impact of the pandemic on the hyper-evolution of digital health care has been well-described. The speed at which digital health has moved means that traditional expectations of larger health systems and organizations have been an ill-affordable luxury for organizations wishing to keep up with the pace of change. This includes processes related to internal development, customization, integration, and triple-line deployment governance. Larger organizations realize the value in helping to grow and distribute as well as incubate innovations, similar to many other industries. Therefore, bringing customers the best possible services requires agility in identifying excellent partners, partnering fairly and promptly, and deploying rapidly.

Customer experience remains paramount of expectations from call center to chairperson. Customer journeys need to be simple, clear, and effective to ensure a great customer experience. A platform for customers can help them explore their needs, understand their options, and access solutions quickly and effectively. A platform can be as simple as a landing page and menu or as complex as an ecosystem linking to a central node which ingests medical records, biometric data, sensor information, and personal communications.

To deliver the right digital health platform for one's business, organizations must consider their option space. The option space digital health can deliver in can vary hugely by the local environment. This spans areas including regulatory expectations, health-system structure, provider readiness, economic position, and patient preferences. Within the option space for partners, organizations must define their vision and then balance the equation of cost, speed, and breadth against this.

At Vitality in the United Kingdom, we recognized the importance of the digital health system early in the last decade, leading us to be the first (and for many years, the only) UK private medical insurer who offered all-inclusive digital primary care access to all of our health insurance customers. All of our eligible customers can access remote musculoskeletal therapy, mental health self-service tools and therapy, care from (hospital-based) specialist physicians, and more. Our evolving Care Hub sits at the heart of this—our suite of digital tools which also allows customers to access and manage details of their insurance policy and supports them to access health care services. In coming years we expect to continue to accelerate how we help customers access high-quality digital health and care support. This is a meaningful business line for us, with quality and outcomes targets and growth expectations— including the over twenty-fold increase in remote care access since we started our journey and the doubling of remote primary care utilization in the first months of 2021.

THOMAS GRANDELL
CEO, Etsimo Healthcare

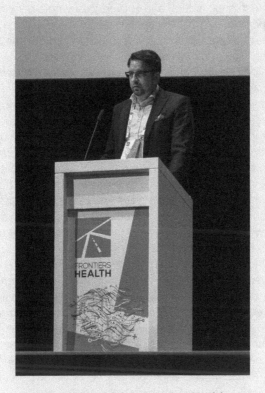

Thomas Grandell at Frontiers Health
Credit: Frontiers Health

Platforms enabling digital health is the future, and the future is almost already here. For such platforms to really provide maximum value, they need to be holistic, and include health resources, digital infrastructure, equipment, facilities, and services to connect and deliver care. In a perfect world, wellness (i.e., nonclinical aspects, also called social determinants of health) that can affect an individual's engagement with their well-being, health, and health care is also included and taken into account. By connecting the dots between patients' circumstances and their health outcomes, we can build targeted interventions that improve patients' physical and mental health and lower the health-care spend.

(Continues)

(*Continued*)

Digital, data-driven solutions make it possible for us to understand the patient in a much greater detail and to produce a whole-person view, paving the way for personalized patient engagements and improved outcomes. In the digital health future, patients are consumers, with both freedom of choice and increasing responsibility for their own health, and this in combination with personalized health insights is the ultimate enabler to removing waste from health-care delivery.

Of the many challenges in building digital health solutions, the major ones have been immature technologies and lack of data (complicated ownership, no interoperability, not sufficiently structured and not in digital format). However, there are currently many initiatives addressing the data issues, and the transformation of health care is being supercharged by three converging technologies: AI, cheap diagnostics (affordable, connected home devices), and always-on health monitoring (wearables). But we must not forget that for digital solutions to work, they need to be built with a consumer-first mindset and be trustworthy—providing easier, faster, better, and cheaper care with empathy, all while keeping the consumers' data safe.

Combining continuous data streams and technology enables instant analysis delivered directly to the consumer or to a care team, anticipating problems before they arise and assisting in providing timely treatments. By utilizing technology, we can reimagine the customer experience, reinvent how we work, and rethink our capabilities so that we provide integrated, consumer-centric, and seamless offerings with better access points and focused care. A future health care where communication/dialogue has moved from transactional to continuous benefits all: the patients, the payers, and the providers.

My company, Etsimo Healthcare Ltd, delivers data-driven health care. We unlock the potential of health data to optimize care needs and provide better care at lower cost. The endgame for us is a learning health system that treats consumer data as fuel in building a continuous whole-person view of the consumer. In other words, in exchange for data, we use a person's past and present to provide insights about their current and future health. This background monitoring of a consumer enables us to react to weak signals, make health predictions and ultimately provide impulses (preventive interventions) to avoid or lower future health risks. Data leads to insights, and insights to more data, and with these capabilities we can shift health care from reactive (i.e., treating sick people) to preventive (i.e., keeping people healthy).

Notes

1. Zenooz, Ashwini M., and John Fox. "How new health care platforms will improve patient care," *Harvard Business Review*, October 11, 2019. Available at: https://hbr.org/2019/10/how-new-health-care-platforms-will-improve-patient-care.
2. Shah, Hiten, and Kiran Kumar. "Ten digital technologies helping humans in the fight against COVID-19," Frost and Sullivan, March 27, 2020. Available at: https://ww2.frost.com/frost-perspectives/ten-digital-technologies-helping-humans-in-the-fight-against-covid-19/.

CHAPTER 6

Digital Therapeutics

A New Phase of Medicine

Can an app replace a drug? The question on the surface may seem rather bizarre. Treating yourself with an app instead of with real medicine isn't a concept that most people are familiar with. Yet, this is the promise of the so-called *digital therapies* (DTx), a term introduced by Roberto Ascione and Marc Slujis, among others. But can software improve people's health the same way that medicine can, cost less, and have no side effects? DTx have been put under the magnifying glass of innovators, researchers, and investors, who foresee vast areas of use of software-based interventions that, tested and studied in the same way that drugs are, offer patients many therapeutic effects. According to the well-known venture capital firm Andreessen Horowitz, a Menlo Park company that invests in innovative startups, digital therapies will be able to advance medicine toward a "third phase," going so far as to complement current drugs that cost billions in production and involve extensive periods of research and development. Looking to the future, Vijay Pande, a doctor and researcher at Stanford University and a partner at Andreessen Horowitz, hypothesized that "the fact that our solution to any health problem is found in a pill will one day seem barbaric and primitive to us." The Digital Therapeutics Alliance, an association founded in 2017 with the aim of fostering greater knowledge and awareness of this sector, defines digital therapies as "evidence-based therapeutic interventions, guided by high-quality software programs to prevent, manage or treat a disorder or medical disease. Not all healthcare apps or technologies are digital therapeutics."

The rise of the digital therapy industry is evidenced by the fact that hundreds of companies are already working in this area, and an increasing number of digital solutions are beginning to produce relevant clinical results, in the same way that traditional clinical practices are doing.

We can recognize two categories of digital therapies. The first is a group of products that behave like dietary supplements and drug adjuvants, while the second type replaces a drug itself. For example, the Sleepio solution developed by Big Health is part of the second group of therapies. Diverse research shows that this digital therapy is more effective than traditional insomnia treatments at helping people sleep better. Researchers developing products in this category make it a point to differentiate themselves from those who work on some of the most common wellness gadgets. To set themselves apart and have a kind of scientific certification, digital therapy companies perform and publish rigorous clinical trials. Sometimes bringing their therapies to market requires authorization from government agencies.

The characteristic feature of these therapies is that they are designed and implemented to focus on the patient's needs. Most of them are related to the treatment of chronic or neurological diseases, which require continuous monitoring. This level of care is often unsustainable for health-care systems and relies on behavioral modification, or lifestyle change in favor of healthier behaviors (e.g., improved nutrition, sleep, movement, etc.). There are already many cases of DTx whose use has had measurable effects on the behavioral change of patients. An example is Somyryst by Pear Therapeutics, digital therapy for chronic insomnia in adults over the age of 22 recognized by the FDA in 2020. In a randomized controlled study of 1,149 Australian adults with insomnia and depressive symptoms, the results indicated that the intervention reduced the amount of time it took to fall asleep by 45 percent, reduced the amount of time spent awake at night by 52 percent, and reduced the severity of the symptoms of insomnia by 45 percent, with continuous improvement at six and 12 months after treatment.[1] And then there's Virta, an app produced by Virta Health in San Francisco, which promises to reverse diabetes without medication or surgery by using online coaching (entrusted to experts in the sector) to induce patients to follow a strict diet that involves a high fat content and a low amount of carbohydrates. It is certainly a very ambitious project that has raised $93 million in funding. A 2019 study showed that Virta's approach reduces the need for prescription drugs. At one year, patients in the clinical trial eliminated 63 percent of diabetes-specific drugs, while 94 percent eliminated or reduced their use of insulin.[2]

In view of the crucial impact on patients in terms of access to care and the sustainability of health-care systems, a growing trend is the increasingly frequent partnerships between companies developing this type of therapy and pharmaceutical companies.

For example, Propeller is no stranger to the pharma space. The company develops products that help people with asthma or chronic obstructive pulmonary disorder (COPD) manage their condition in partnership with their health-care provider. In 2017, Propeller has already made deals with GlaxoSmithKline and more recently has teamed up with Novartis to co-package the digital health platform for their asthma medication, so that Propeller's sensors can collect medication data and send that information to a corresponding app. The tool works both as an adherence measure, giving the patient reminders to take their medication, and as a means of collecting information about the patient's condition.

Despite the many benefits that DTx can have on the sustainability of health systems, the international scene of digital therapies is still very fragmented, curbing the growth and widespread dissemination of this new generation of therapies in the various global healthcare systems. The United States proves to be the most dynamic context, in that the Federal Drug Administration (FDA) for several years has considered DTx as true healing interventions, thus determining their availability and possibility for reimbursement. In Europe, it is important to highlight the momentum given to digital therapies by German Parliament's 2019 decision to authorize their use (as they did for other digital tools with important scientific evidence)[3] and to allow their reimbursement by insurance companies. This makes Germany one of the first countries to reimburse digital health solutions systematically and broadly through public insurance, allowing 73 million people in Germany to get a free digital health app prescribed by a doctor.

However, the presence or absence of implementation or reimbursement models does not imply that DTx has already entered fully into the medical practice. In fact, there are many factors that hinder its actual adoption. Some barriers are linked to the specific nature of this innovation while others are attributable to the health-care professionals, institutions, and patients.

Roberto's Vision

We are surrounded by a huge number of platforms that store our data and have value and applicability in the health field. It is as if each of us had a series of projections of our habits and behaviors that, taken as a whole, constitute an information sphere of our state of health, or even of our clinical condition. When we have all this information at our disposal, we may also decide to integrate it, to authorize other information systems to process it, and to obtain information useful for a wide range of processes in return. At the present time, the data is very often unstructured, hybridized, and from different platforms. It is also not easy to cross-reference. The great development of artificial intelligence (AI) applications on this type of data is very important because it makes it possible to extrapolate information that otherwise could not be processed with more conventional algorithms.

We can see this period of intense transformation as the dawn of digital health or the continuation of digital health. In the future we ourselves could be carrying a great number of sensors that passively record information. For example, today there are apps for the control of eating habits in which one must manually enter everything eaten during the day. Even for those most dedicated to entering their data, this methodology, in the long run, is not sustainable. It would be much more interesting, however, if the dish one is using understood on its own what you are eating and in what quantities and down-loaded the calorie intake independently and automatically onto one of these platforms. Let's imagine a world dominated by sensors that collect this information, consolidate it into integration systems (e.g., Apple's Health Kit, or other types of platforms), analyze the data, and return feedback on it. They could tell us, "Get up and exercise," "Eat more," or "Eat less," and of course, some elements could become even more sophisticated. Amicomed, an Italian-Swiss startup is one of these platforms. It is dedicated to those who have problems with blood pressure. A patient's pressure values are communicated to the app which, using a sophisticated algorithm, identifies what the person's pressure profile is. The app then draws up a daily diet program for 90 days, with advice on physical activity and with bits of useful information. A study conducted by the American College of Cardiology and the American Hypertension Society showed that after 90 days of the app's use, blood pressure dropped, on average, by five millimeters of mercury, not an insignificant figure when you consider that there has been no pharmacological intervention. Of course, this does not mean that use of Amicomed will fully replace a blood-pressure pill, but one can use this app to prevent a certain problem, or combine it with diet and/or a drug therapy. Perhaps Amicomed could require lower drug dosages or fewer medications in combination.

There are many other applications, some that are already used by millions of people, including those that focus on diabetes. Using DTx to support behavior modification is certainly a very promising trend. On the way are more software-driven interventions that have a measurable and scientifically validated clinical impact. For example, a collaboration between Kaiku Health and Roche is aimed at co-developing new digital patient monitoring and management modules in oncology. Another, developed by Sidekick Health and Pfizer, uses gamification to offer patients a new support tool for maintaining healthy lifestyles, while providing guidance and resources to facilitate easier and faster communication with their healthcare professionals.

The idea is to be able to perform actions using a method based on these algorithms or even classically. It is important to remember that the fundamental theme remains the implementation of digital solutions in clinical practice, and to this end, the launch of strategic partnerships plays a central and strategic role.

Akili

Akili Interactive, a U.S. company in the DTx industry, is a pioneer in the development of digital treatments for therapeutic purposes delivered not through a pill, but through a high-quality gaming experience. Thanks to continuous research in the field, collaboration with world-renowned cognitive neuroscientists, and experienced entertainment and technology designers, Akili has built a wide range of programs for treating cognitive impairment and improving symptoms associated with medical conditions in neurology and psychiatry. The digital medicine created by Akili, EndeavorRx (AKL-T01), has been approved by the FDA and today is the first video game recognized as digital therapy for children with attention deficit/hyperactivity disorder (ADHD).

Delivered through a captivating video game experience, EndeavorRx is indicated to improve attention function as measured by computer-based testing in children ages eight to 12 years old with primarily inattentive or combined-type ADHD, who have a demonstrated attention issue.

EndeavorRx was granted clearance based on data from five clinical studies in more than 600 children diagnosed with ADHD, including a prospective, randomized, controlled study published in *The Lancet Digital Health* journal, which showed EndeavorRx improved objective measures of attention in children with ADHD. After four weeks of EndeavorRx treatment, one-third of children no longer had a measurable attention deficit on at least one measure of objective attention. Further, about half of parents saw a clinically meaningful change in their child's day-to-day impairments after one month of treatment with EndeavorRx; this increased to 68 percent after a second month of treatment. Improvements in ADHD impairments following a month of treatment with EndeavorRx were maintained for up to a month.

Akili is also committed to developing digital treatments for people with autism, depression, Alzheimer's disease, and head trauma. In a study conducted with Pfizer, for example, the use of Akili's technology has shown that it can detect the biomarkers of Alzheimer's disease.

Amicomed

Amicomed is an Italian startup based in Switzerland and Italy that has developed a digital service for the management of blood pressure via lifestyle changes rather than medications. The smartphone app is designed for hypertensive persons based on the needs of users. It has been designed to improve blood pressure values by promoting lifestyle improvements based on diet and movement with the help of motivational triggers and a pleasant and intuitive interface. The program proposed by Amicomed has a duration of three months and allows people to control hypertension by providing professional advice on what foods they should be eating, what type of physical activity they should be doing, and how and when they should measure their blood pressure. In a nutshell, it is an innovative coaching program, curated by doctors, nutritionists, and sport-science experts. In addition, of course, IT technicians collaborate to develop complex algorithms that allow the provision of the service.

Amicomed relies on Quasarmed, an Italian company that has developed and owns the Pascal algorithm, the first that is dedicated to the interpretation of blood pressure that has also been certified as a medical device. Amicomed does not intend to replace doctors, but rather it wants to be an aid and a support that allows the health-care professional to better analyze the patient's condition in order to achieve a more precise diagnosis and thus optimally calibrate a possible therapy. Amicomed is also useful for people without a particular pathology because it can help those who are healthy to evaluate their situation in a simple and reliable way, preventing the establishment of hypertensive phenomena. During 2016 the excellent results obtained by the app were studied by numerous international universities and considered scientifically relevant, so much so that they were also presented at the main medical congresses such as the American College of Cardiology and the American Society of Hypertension. Thanks to the positive results obtained with the first tests in Italy, Amicomed was the only European company selected by Launchpad Digital Health—Ground Zero (LDHGZ), the first and so far the only business accelerator that aims at integrating new entrepreneurs into its innovative digital health hub, a digital space where resources for innovation and ideas for developing new solutions and new entrepreneurship in the field of health are intertwined.

Click Therapeutics

Click Therapeutics is a biotechnology company that develops, validates, and commercializes software as prescription medical treatments for people with unmet medical needs. It entered a collaboration with key pharma player Boehringer Ingelheim to develop and commercialize a novel prescription digital therapeutic (CT-155) to aid in the treatment of schizophrenia.

Through cognitive and neurobehavioral mechanisms, Click's Digital Therapeutics enable change within individuals, and are designed to be used independently or in conjunction with biomedical treatments. The adaptive data-science platform implemented by Click, The Clickometrics, continuously personalizes the user experience to optimize engagement and outcomes. Based on the results of dedicated clinical trials, Click launched a smoking cessation program in the United States through a wide variety of payers, providers, and employers. The company is progressing a broad pipeline of DTx across a variety of high-burden therapeutic areas, including major depressive disorder, acute coronary syndrome, chronic pain, insomnia, COPD, obesity, and more.

Ginger.io

Founded in 2010 in the MIT Media Lab, Ginger initially developed a platform that collected information from mobile phones to alert patients (and if necessary, their attending physicians) when they were affected by manic behavior, or if there had been a general worsening of an already debilitating disease.

Today Ginger has developed a digital mental health service that provides services of coaching, video therapy, telepsychiatry visits, and other mental health support activities. In particular, it is aimed at people who suffer from depression and anxiety or who need emotional support.

The World Economic Forum identified Ginger's AI technology as a Technology Pioneer, and it was recognized as one of the 10 most innovative companies in the health-care industry by *Fast Company*. In August 2021, Ginger merged with Headspace to provide a full range of mental health services to their customers, demonstrating the importance of providing full continuum from prevention/wellness to care.

Kaia Health

Kaia Health was founded by Manuel Thurner and Konstantin Mehl in 2015, when they united in their mission to find a more effective way for managing chronic back pain. Today they offer programs to help people with chronic back pain and COPD. Kaia Health started with a digital physiotherapy platform for back pain, which guides users through exercises at home, thus proposing its technology as an alternative to traditional analgesics. Through its app, Kaia aims at empowering and motivating patients to self-manage their condition with digital alternatives from their home using devices that they already own. Thanks to its clinically validated technology, every smartphone can become a digital personal trainer or physiotherapist capable of analyzing the human body and offering instructions and feedback in real time.

The company is still focused on treating musculoskeletal disorders; however, it is rapidly expanding its range of services so as to include exercise and wellness tools and treatment programs for the symptoms of COPD. The platform has served over 400,000 users in just four years since its launch and today it is the world's most widely used global digital therapeutic platform.

Voluntis

Voluntis, a French company with headquarters in Paris, is active in the development of therapeutic support software for doctors and patients. One of the digital therapy solutions it has developed concerns patients with diabetes. It is a software that can support patients throughout their insulin therapy treatment. Insulia (this is the name of the digital product) is a solution for people with Type 2 diabetes in treatment with long-acting basal insulin. The software provides patients with insulin dose recommendations and informative coaching messages.

In addition to Insulia, Voluntis has developed similar digital solutions for the treatment of respiratory diseases, cancer, and hemophilia. For example, Oleena is the first FDA-approved second-class medical device to be marketed for use in all indications related to various types of cancer. Oleena is an app that allows cancer patients to self-manage their symptoms and keep under control the common side effects that they experience. Thanks to a connected portal, it also favors remote monitoring and support by the medical team.

Guest Perspectives

EUGENE BORUKHOVICH
Chairman & COO YourCoach Health

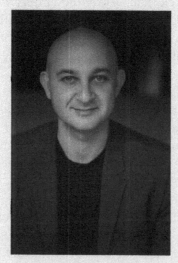

Eugene Borukhovich
Credit: Eugene Boruchovich – Private archive

In the ever-expanding promise of the digital health industry lies the shining light of "medical interventions directly to patients using evidence-based, clinically evaluated software to treat, manage, and prevent a broad spectrum of diseases and disorders." (That is the official definition by the consortium of companies under the Digital Therapeutics Alliance (DTA).) While the term *digital therapeutics* was coined sometime in 2012, it was not until the DTA came onto the scene in 2017, combined with early clinical evidence from many trailblazers in the industry, that the abbreviation DTx started to really take shape. While still at the early stages of mass adoption, these technologies hold the promise of democratizing access to health and care. This new, data-driven modality is starting to take shape around the world, from the United States to Belgium to South Korea, but it is also starting to quickly evolve into a multitude of go-to-market approaches, be it prescription-only, over the counter, or completely new and virtual service models that encapsulate a DTx as part of the experience. I ultimately see the term *digital* disappearing and leaving therapeutic as yet another set of tools in the arsenal.

We saw healthcare systems around the world almost crumble during the pandemic; governments around the world responded, some better than others. As an example, the FDA, in an unprecedented move in April 2020, expanded " . . . the availability of digital health therapeutic devices for psychiatric disorders to facilitate consumer and patient use . . ."[4] I do believe this will drive the much-needed awareness, adoption and even more clinical outcomes for digital therapies going forward—consider this the silver lining of the pandemic.

As a society, we have never paid more attention to our own health and health of our loved ones but establishing those health goals and having the drive to reach them is very much tied to our behaviors. Our mission at YourCoach Health is for every person on this planet to have access to a squad of health and wellness coaches, the new frontlines of health. We strongly believe that the human eye to this day and for the foreseeable future will continue to be better than AI but this nascent workforce of individuals, armed with science-backed and behavior-driven approaches, will be leading the way. There is no better complement than self-paced therapeutic technologies in a health coach's "health scribing" arsenal to help people—to help us be happy humans and live healthier and happier lives.

(*Continues*)

(*Continued*)

MEGAN CODER
PharmD, MBA; Executive Director, Digital Therapeutics Alliance

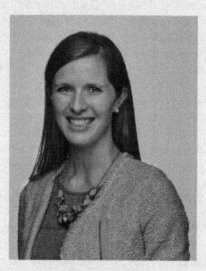

Megan Coder
Credit: Megan Coder – Private archive

When building a home, it is necessary to start with a strong foundation. When building an industry, the same notion applies. Since 2017, the Digital Therapeutics Alliance (DTA) has therefore focused on constructing the necessary foundation for the rapidly evolving DTx industry.

To ensure that all stakeholders have a common way to recognize and understand this new category of products, we first collectively developed an industry-accepted definition of a digital therapeutic. Next, to ensure that all DTx products across the industry demonstrate a consistent, reliable level of quality, safety, and efficacy, we built a series of 10 principles that all products ought to meet in order to qualify as a digital therapeutic.

From there, we added to this foundation by developing an industry code of ethics, a framework to differentiate DTx products from other digital health tools, and a matrix for stakeholders to distinguish between various DTx product types within the category. With the understanding that the future of healthcare will unquestionably include products that generate and deliver medical interventions directly to patients using software to treat, manage, and prevent diseases and disorders, it is now our role to build on this foundation and develop much-needed framing for the industry. The sooner that policy-makers, payors, clinicians, and patients want to see these products scaled and integrated into healthcare systems, the more urgently these critical obstacles must be addressed and overcome:

- **Policymakers.** First, policymakers require a framework to categorize DTx products based on intended use and risk. In the coming years, we expect a globally consistent pathway to market to emerge, with the recognition that nations will layer-in additional country-specific clinical and economic outcome requirements.
- **Payers.** Second, we foresee that a cohesive framework for payors will be developed to evaluate and cover DTx products. Without consistent requirements of clinical trial data, real-world outcomes, and data governance requirements, DTx product scalability across local, regional, and national systems will be greatly limited, potentially depriving entire populations of access to new therapies.
- **Clinicians and patients.** Lastly, clinicians, patients, and caregivers face steep learning curves in understanding what digital therapeutics are and how to appropriately use them and extract the greatest value. In the coming years, clinical guidelines related to the appropriate use of DTx products, technical training for optimizing product use, and patient-centric support for integrating digital therapeutics into daily lifestyles will be developed.

Given the global need to address growing mental health concerns, provide remote care for patients with chronic conditions, and enhance healthcare delivery processes, it is crucial that over the coming years we proactively work together to address current gaps in care and provide patients with access to evidence-based digital therapeutics.

Notes

1. Pear Therapeutics. "Pear Therapeutics announces data from two studies evaluating Somryst™ for chronic insomnia presented at Virtual SLEEP 2020," press release, n.d. Available at: https://peartherapeutics.com/pear-therapeutics-announces-data-from-two-studies-evaluating-somryst-for-chronic-insomnia-presented-at-virtual-sleep-2020/.

2. Virta Health. "Outcomes," VirtaHealth.com, n.d. Available at: https://www.virtahealth.com/outcomes.
3. Bundesministerium für Gesundheit. "Ärzte sollen Apps verschreiben können," n.d. Available at: https://www.bundesgesundheitsministerium.de/digitale-versorgung-gesetz.html.
4. U.S. Food and Drug Administration. "Enforcement policy for digital health devices for treating psychiatric disorders during the coronavirus disease 2019 (COVID-19) public health emergency," FDA Guidance Document, April 2020. Available at: https://www.fda.gov/regulatory-information/search-fda-guidance-documents/enforcement-policy-digital-health-devices-treating-psychiatric-disorders-during-coronavirus-disease.

Personal Genomics

From Mendel to Portable DNA Mapping Machines

It has been a while since an Augustinian monk named Gregor Mendel conducted his experiments on pea plants, drawing ingenious deductions. It was 1866 when his *Experiments on Plant Hybrids* was printed, a text that was understood by very few people at the time, but which can now be considered as one of the cornerstones of genetics. To have the certainty that genetic information is contained within DNA, and to also solve the many doubts about the shape of this strange molecule present in the nucleus of cells, it was necessary to wait until 1953. Thanks to James Watson and Francis Crick, we now know its double-helix shape gives DNA its distinct appearance. The successive studies in 1968 by Har Gobid Khorana, Robert W. Holley, and Marshall W. Nirenberg then allowed the code to be deciphered, laying the foundations of modern genetics and molecular biology. And many more years would come to pass before the completion of the so-called Human Genome Project (HGP), an international scientific research project whose main objective was identifying and mapping the human genome from a physical and functional point of view. The work, which lasted more than a decade, was completed on June 24, 2003. The DNA sequence, as is widely known, contains all the hereditary genetic information. Within this sequence are encoded the genes of each living organism, as well as the instructions for expressing them in time and space. Determining the sequence is therefore useful for understanding how biological systems work and the way they interact with the environment. Over time, several strategies have been devised in order to obtain the nucleotide of the DNA sequence.

The first methods are dated 1973. This includes the rather complicated procedure designed by Allan Maxam and Walter Gilbert. In 1975, there was an improvement in Maxam and Gilbert's methods, coming from the enzymatic method designed by Frederick Sanger (the so-called *chain termination method* or *Sanger method*), for which he received the Nobel Prize. A turning point in the sequencing techniques, thanks to the use of innovative technologies with a high production capacity, able to simultaneously perform an incredibly high quantity of sequencing, even of the order of billions, took place at the beginning of the century. They have been called technologies with *high-level parallelism*, thanks to their characteristic ability to sequence so many things at once. This evolution led to the birth and development of many technologies grouped under the name of next-generation sequencing (NGS), a series of methodologies that make it possible to sequence large parts of a genome in a short time, generally, a few days. The use of these innovative techniques makes it possible, in a single experiment, to carry out various types of studies, including the simultaneous characterization of genomes, the identification of balanced and unbalanced chromosomal rearrangements, deletions, and more.

The year 2018 opened with an extraordinary announcement in this field. The team of Nicholas Loman of the University of Birmingham and Matthew Loose of the University of Nottingham developed a portable mapping device for sequencing portions of the human genome. This device was able to provide data with exceptional speed, high accuracy, and at a low cost, allowing the team to then analyze this data for the rapid development of appropriate therapies. The device, named MinION, was produced by a company called Oxford Nanopore. It involves the passage of long strands of DNA into a minuscule hole, called a *nanopore*, and the final result of sequencing boasts, according to the researchers, an accuracy rate of 99.88 percent. As Loman himself explained to the BBC online: "We've gone from a situation where you can only do genome sequencing for a huge amount of money in well-equipped labs to one where we can have genome sequencing literally in your pocket just like a mobile phone. That gives us a really exciting opportunity to start having genome sequencing as a routine tool, perhaps something people can do in their own home."[1] A MinION technology has the potential of changing medicine and diagnostics as we now know it. The future has already begun.

In 2020, the Virology Laboratory of the National Institute for Infectious Diseases in Rome (*Lazzaro Spallanzani*) was among the very first in Europe to generate sequencing data of the entire genome of the novel coronavirus SARS-CoV-2.

"Thanks to the high-resolution power achieved with this type of NGS sequencing, we are able to analyze the presence of even minority variants that are generated during viral replication. Generally, this is not possible with other massive sequencing approaches (e.g., shotgun), since coverage along the genome is not uniform and a very high viral load is required to achieve complete and informative sequencing,"[2] said Dr. Capobianchi, Director of the Institute's Virology Laboratory.

The timely availability of sequences in the international GISAID database has been crucial in tracking the evolutionary trajectory of the virus, in the individuation of possible pathogenic variants and, above all, in identifying the targets for the vaccine, which was then developed and made available since the end of the year.

Roberto's Vision

The opportunities that are being developed in this area are due to the combination of a series of relatively recent innovations which, operating together, are opening up new avenues for action for the improvement of the health of each one of us. In this field, aspects relating to genetic research in the strict sense intersect with aspects of advanced informatics, technology, computer science, and of digital technology in a more general sense. Let's take a look at the reasons one by one, starting with genetics, in the strict sense. Obviously, at the beginning of this revolution there are the sequencing techniques that have made it possible, over the years, to obtain a complete mapping of the human genome. These methods have developed up to the so-called NGS, the current DNA sequencing techniques, the cost of which has seen a sharp decrease. It will swiftly go from a few thousand dollars to a few hundred dollars to sequence a single person's DNA. The possibility of sequencing complete DNA at an extremely affordable cost makes this type of large-scale practice possible even today (and it will be even more so in the near future), creating a first, very useful database level. In reality, as a source of data there is not only DNA sequencing (i.e., genomics), but also proteomics (i.e., the large-scale study of proteins, in particular their structures and functions), microbiomics (the mapping of all the microorganisms that inhabit our intestines), and metabolomics (the study of the metabolites produced by specific cellular processes). Each of these studies generates an incredibly vast amount of data, with primarily unstructured and complex levels of information. To make the picture even more articulated, we can add all the images produced with the various CT scans, MRIs, ultrasounds, x-rays, and so on. This provides a further wealth of information that is also unstructured. Finally, we have all the information related to other data, such as the results of blood and urine tests and so on. If we seek to be complete, we can add other unstructured information, including data collected by various smart devices that track what we eat, how much we drink, how much we move, how much pressure we use when we type on the smartphone keypad, and a wealth of other datapoints.

This information is apparently unrelated to the health-care domain, but it is of enormous value. Why? Because most pathological conditions develop as a result of the interaction between a specific genetic predisposition and an entire series of environmental factors (related precisely to lifestyle, nutrition, movement, sedentary lifestyle, and so on) that revolve around the DNA itself, determining whether or not it is expressed. And now we have come to the technological side of the question: this set of data (the DNA mapping, all the other biological systems, other behavioral information tracked by other types of sensors) comprise a huge mass of information that is largely, as mentioned, unstructured. But the development of next-generation algorithms able to handle huge amounts of data is about to put an end to this chaos. These algorithms, referred to as machine learning (ML) (and which are part of the large family of data science or artificial intelligence (AI), as it is commonly called), are not responsible for performing a sequence of predefined instructions, but are able to work substantially in reverse, that is, finding correlations between the huge amount of data they analyze and the behaviors that are in some way related to them. Imagine that we have a vast amount of data available on a large number of individuals. The goal is for each of these individuals to know whether or not the diagnosis related to their pathologies is confirmed. Algorithms can be used to compare and identify correlations between two things, going even further than the objectives for which they were programmed (hence the concept of ML). In essence, the machine finds correlations and offers them, very quickly, to an analyst doctor as suggestions to be verified. The availability of this category of algorithms, and the ability to collect and store large amounts of data at an ever-lower cost, is paving the way for increasingly early diagnosis and the possibility of preventing a series of conditions that, until now, we could not imagine were related to a certain type of pathological condition. That is how a horizon of great possibilities has opened up. In the case of complex pathologies, such as tumors, this technique will increasingly provide the possibility of having hyper-personalized treatments on the individual and on the individual type of tumor that the person has contracted, making it possible to select the most effective drug in that specific condition and thus avoiding a series of other treatments that would be ineffective or partially effective (if not, in fact, harmful). All this is possible thanks to the convergence between sequencing technologies and big data processing technologies. On the prevention front, the possibility of identifying a genetic susceptibility, and therefore, an increase in the probability of developing a certain type of condition and having the possibility of correlating the development of this possible pathology with a series of behaviors that can be implemented, allows a completely innovative prevention strategy that in past times could not go beyond general behavioral advice. The revolution, in this sense, will be substantial. We will move from the current approach to prevention, which is based on generic suggestions of correct lifestyles, to something extremely personalized, with very specific interventions whose ultimate aim will be to delay (or even avoid) the onset of pathologies.

23andMe

23andMe is a private company co-founded by Anne Wojcicki, ex-wife of Sergey Brin (who, together with Larry Page, created Google), that deals with genomics and biotechnology, with headquarters in Mountain View, California. In 2008, her saliva-based genetic collection and analysis was named "Invention of the Year" by *Time* magazine. Thanks to this test, it is possible to reveal whether or not a person is at risk for a series of diseases: Parkinson's disease, Alzheimer's, celiac disease, alpha1 antitrypsin deficiency (disease that increases the risk of lung and liver diseases), primary dystonia (movement disorder), factor XI deficiency (blood clotting disorder), Gaucher's disease, glucose-6-phosphate dehydrogenase deficiency (G6PD), hereditary hemochromatosis (iron overload disorder), hereditary thrombophilia, and Type 2 diabetes.

The authorization of 23andMe tests was supported by data from the scientific literature that demonstrated a link between specific genetic variants and each of these pathologies. The tests provide information on genetic risk, but obviously, they cannot take into account all the other factors that come into play in determining whether or not a person will fall ill with a particular disease. All the company's tests were carried out on a saliva sample tested for more than 500,000 genetic variants. The company's database contains over a million genetic profiles, a resource considered very valuable by numerous pharmaceutical companies. "Consumers can now have direct access to certain genetic risk information," explains Jeffrey Shuren, director of the FDA's Center for Devices and Radiological Health, "but it's important that they understand how genetic risk is just one piece of a much larger puzzle." In fact, the risk of developing a specific disease can be determined by diverse environmental factors and lifestyle as much as by genetics. Tests should not be used to make a diagnosis, but to help consumers make decisions about lifestyle choices to adopt or to allow them to discuss these choices with their doctor.

Deep Genomics

Deep Genomics, founded in 2015, is located in the heart of Toronto, the fastest-growing technology hub in North America and one of the world's most livable cities. It has facilities ranging from experimental biology to computational analysis, and is located near the University of Toronto, four research hospitals, three medical research institutes and the research laboratories of Google, Uber, and Vector. A nice place for a meeting of minds! The conviction of Deep Genomics is that the future of medicine will be based on the use of AI because, as they say, the biology is too complex to be understood by humans. The molecular structure of a cell can be investigated experimentally like never before, and the resulting datasets provide an unprecedented opportunity for building AI systems that are biologically accurate and support disease detection and the development of molecular interventions. Deep Genomics is building a biologically accurate platform based on this type of data and AI to support geneticists, molecular biologists, and chemists in the development of therapies. It uses IA to support every stage of drug development, from identifying therapeutic targets, which had previously been omitted as nonpharmacologically viable, to designing new therapeutic candidates, to designing animal models. The approach translates into remarkable clarity and speed. Seventy percent of research projects have led to therapeutic results, and the programs have been brought from the discovery of the target to the drug candidate in less than 12 months.

Deep Genomics' goal is using its platform to unlock new classes of antisense oligonucleotidic therapies that complement a given sequence and advance it for clinical evaluation. Antisense oligonucleotides are small, single-stranded molecules of DNA or RNA. As cofounder Brendan Frey pointed out, "In the vision of Deep Genomics, the pharmaceutical company of the future will resemble a computer company, with an incredible team of biologists, chemists, and experts in clinical and non-clinical trials, unlike a traditional pharmaceutical company with biologists and chemists using IT tools. It's a matter of culture, a culture of computer science."

Flatiron Health

Nat Turner and Zach Weinberg founded Flatiron Health in 2012, shortly after their first company (Invite Media, an online advertising company) was purchased by Google. Flatiron's idea had already been circulating in the minds of the two founders for a few years. Turner's seven-year-old cousin Brennan was diagnosed with a rare form of leukemia. During Brennan's treatment, Turner and Weinberg realized how fragmented and inefficient the health-care system was. Based on this experience, in order to transform the way cancer is studied and treated, their idea was to bring together some of the best minds in medicine and technology. Flatiron harnesses the potential of digital technology to collect clinical data from cancer patients: what drugs they have taken or are taking, how they have responded to various medicines and dosages, what side effects they have recorded, and so on.

Flatiron's goal is to make sure that doctors can build a better idea of how cancer drugs work in the "real world," that is, in hospitals and cancer centers, rather than during clinical trials. The company raised more than $300 million from investors including GV and the pharmaceutical giant Roche, which acquired Flatiron in February 2018 at a cost of about $2 billion. The experience of every cancer patient is extremely important, and each patient's story has the unique potential to teach something new about the way cancer acts. This information can help to discover the most effective treatments more quickly. Flatiron's team believes that learning from these experiences is the key to accelerating research and continuing to improve the quality of care. Today, most of the available clinical data is unstructured and stored in thousands of clinics, medical centers, and hospitals, all of them disconnected from each other. That is a problem that Flatiron seeks to solve. Currently, Flatiron collaborates with 280 cancer clinics, seven major academic research centers, and more than 15 of the most relevant therapeutic oncology companies in the United States.

Human Longevity

Human Longevity is a company founded in San Diego in 2013 and offers comprehensive genome analysis and other sophisticated diagnostic tests such as bone densimetry, MRI tomography, and CT scans for identifying abnormalities that could lead to the onset of disease or even premature death. The company, founded by renowned scientist Craig Venter and Peter Diamandis, aims at slowing down the human ageing process through a better understanding of people's genetic heritage. The basic idea that led to the establishment of the Human Longevity project is a clinical service based on a remarkable paradigm shift. Today we care about health only when we are sick or when the first symptoms of a disease manifest themselves. Human Longevity, however, is able to provide proactive health-care assistance when a person is still healthy, so that they treat certain conditions that a person is unaware of having. Human Longevity combines its database of genomic and phenotype data with machine learning to drive the discoveries and revolutionize the practice of medicine. In 2020, Human Longevity published the study "Precision medicine integrating whole-genome sequencing, comprehensive metabolomics, and advanced imaging" demonstrating how genome sequencing makes it possible to identify the potential risk of chronic diseases in adult patients. "The goal of precision medicine is to provide a path to assist physicians in achieving disease prevention and implementing accurate treatment strategies," said C. Thomas Caskey, Chief Medical Officer of Human Longevity, lead author of the study, and member of the National Academy of Sciences. "Our study has shown that by using a holistic, data-driven health assessment for each individual, we are able to get an early diagnosis of the disease in adults."

Sophia Genetics

Sophia Genetics is a Swiss company founded in 2011 that operates in the field of clinical genomics. Thanks to the adoption of digital technologies, such as next-generation DNA sequencing (NGS), Sophia Genetics has entered the world of big data. In order to successfully analyze the huge amount of sequenced data, the team of experts of Sophia Genetics has developed Sophia AI, a universal technology that is already used today by over 990 health-care institutions worldwide, each of which brings its own contribution to the Sophia Genetics genomic community through data-driven medicine (DDM). Sophia AI takes advantage of statistical inferences, pattern recognition, and machine learning to maximize the value of genomic and radiomic data.

By reading a patient's entire genomic sequence, it helps doctors diagnose a wide range of diseases.

Precisely through the tools made available by Sophia Genetics, a large number of experts can interpret the data more easily and quickly, evaluate their variations, mark them with the appropriate level of pathogenicity, and share the acquired knowledge with other members of the community. The extraordinary result of this large-scale collaboration is the possibility it gives doctors around the world for finding the best treatment options for their patients.

Cellarity

Founded in 2017 by Flagship Pioneering, Cellarity focuses on the complex networks embedded in every cell and the potential for computation to target the full complexity of disease biology to accelerate medical breakthroughs. The Flagship team envisioned that those technologies could generate the data needed to unravel biological complexity. In short, Cellarity has built a platform to discover and develop medicines by studying and altering cell behaviors to dramatically increase the success rate and speed for drug discovery.[3]

Guest Perspective

OSCAR FLORES
Co-Founder and CEO, Made of Genes

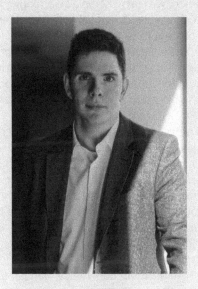

Oscar Flores

Credit: Oscar Flores

When we talk about "personal genomics" we usually think about direct-to-consumer genetic tests (DTC-GT). Today, 15 years after the foundation of 23andMe, the worldwide referent of DTC-GT which has grown at double-digit rate during this period, we can observe from the 2020s a slow-down in the adoption rate of its demand, in part coupled to the emergence of competitors, the saturation of the early-adopters niche, and the fact that they are mostly curiosity-driven tests lacking a delivery of real value besides learning about one's ancestors.

A signal that DTC-GT is not a really promising sector is the fact that, despite 23andMe's announcing its multibillion-dollar IPO in 2021, there is no other pure DTC-GT company in the landscape that is expected to soon reach

(*Continues*)

(Continued)

this milestone. The closest company is MyHeritage, which is clearly focused in the curiosity-driven ancestry branch. Even Veritas Genomics, the company that once was multi-awarded by their promise of sequencing and keeping end-customers' whole genomes (Veritas Genomics was co-founded by George Church, a pioneer of personalized medicine and genetics professor at Harvard Medical School and MIT).

In the meantime, DTC-GT is struggling to find a consumer's niche. During the same period, we can observe a booming in the molecular diagnosis sector. Same technique, different value. Tens or even hundreds of companies valued over or close to $1 billion have emerged in recent years such as Guardant Health, Foundation Medicine or Invitae, proving that competence is not a problem when the solved pain is real. These companies do not rely on the willingness of end-customers to pay for a test to sate their curiosity, but on the real need of health-care professionals to diagnose, treat, or prevent diseases.

And between these two worlds, we find myriad companies that offer non-clinical health-care services based on genetics, such as nutrigenomics or personalized training plans. *A priori*, it seems that this approach should work, because a lot of end-customers are already paying to have a nutritionist plan a diet or a trainer supervise their sports routines. But, again, we face the same problem of curiosity-driven ancestry test: the lack of actionability. Clinical genomics provide actionable findings and are regulated by health-care supervisors. DTC-GT applied to health care are not. With the current low-cost techniques, DNA sampling kits and public know-how available, a company can launch an at-home non-clinical genetic test in less than one month with a cost less than a few thousand dollars. There is no real barrier to the unregulated sector, and the low-hanging fruit of uneducated users not knowing what they are purchasing is too attractive for ethically relaxed companies.

Only with the use of genetics can we diagnose, assess risks, or predict individual outcomes for a few diseases. However, what can be useful in disease management is not applicable to health management. Using only genetics, we cannot assess or improve our present or future general health status as the weight of environmental factors ranges between 70 and 90 percent, depending on the condition. Despite genetics once being presented as the crystal ball that would forecast our future health, today we know it is just another relevant data point of our overall health biology.

In my opinion, the future of this field called *personal genomics* is no longer based on genomics, but will be described as "personalized health-care using molecular studies." This is what we are pursuing at Made of Genes: using objective and quantifiable molecular information—related to genomics, epigenomics, metabolomics, microbiome, and so on—combined with digital health-care techniques—such as systems biology, bioinformatics, and artificial intelligence—we aim to perform high-precision assessments of a current user's health and provide actionable recommendations about how to improve habits to revert or control altered status.

This approach is way more complicated than just crossing gene alleles with a database to retrieve a statistic, and probably biased, risk, but it works. At Made of Genes we observed—and our health-care partners witnessed—that this approach is capable of delivering a real value to both patients and professionals, even not being a traditional IVD clinical genetic test focused on disease management. At the end of the day, this is where the final challenge of personalized medicine is: shifting the current paradigm of health care from disease management to health preservation.

Notes

1. Gallagher, James. "Handheld device sequences human genome," BBC News, January 29, 2018. Available at: https://www.bbc.com/news/health-42838821.
2. Panorama della Sanita. "Covid-19: Dalle nuove tecniche di sequenziamento del genoma virale un importante contributo ad una maggiore conoscenza del virus," *Studi e Ricerca*, March 27, 2020. Available at: https://www.panoramasanita.it/2020/03/27/covid-19-dalle-nuove-tecniche-di-sequenziamento-del-genoma-virale-un-importante-contributo-ad-una-maggiore-conoscenza-del-virus/.
3. Cellarity. "About," Cellarity.com, n.d. Available at: https://cellarity.com/about.

CHAPTER 8

Open Innovation and Partnerships

How Companies Are Moving: The Speed and Intuition of Smaller Companies

For more than a decade, the traditional model of company innovation has entered a state of crisis. Until the beginning of the new millennium, the traditional model was one of the main ones with which a company could build an advantage in the market vis-à-vis other competing companies. What does this innovation strategy consist of? Here is a summary of the innovation scenario: The tendency of large companies, until just recently, was to carry out innovation within the perimeter of their own walls, creating ad hoc research and development structures in order to gain an advantage over the competition: everything that was conceived and created was owned by the company and nothing could escape into the outside world. This way of doing innovation was later renamed *closed innovation*. The recent fluidity of the world of work has, however, led to the evolution of a new way of doing innovation. We have therefore moved from closed innovation to one that is open. The definition of *open innovation* comes from Henry Chesbrough, who currently serves as director of the Center for Open Innovation at the Haas School of Business at the University of California. Chesbrough first described open innovation in his book *The Era of Open Innovation*. The cornerstone of the reasoning was that large research and development centers run by corporations were no longer efficient structures for innovating and remaining competitive in ever-accelerating markets. In fact, closed innovation produces a real advantage only when certain conditions are met (i.e., when the working group within the company is large enough and well trained so as to have the capacity to develop products with a certain continuity). If this condition does not occur, the advantage does not materialize, and the most practical, and decidedly most profitable, solution for a company to create an information flow that can lead to more ambitious goals is to look outside, involving prepared and motivated startups, university work groups, or institutions.

Rivers of ink have flowed concerning the goodness of open innovation, and there is no shortage of examples of how this type of approach has contributed to the success of many large companies (e.g., Apple, Google, and Netflix) and has instead condemned those who, in a short-sighted way, had remained anchored in the old paradigms of innovation (e.g., Kodak, Nokia, and BlackBerry to name the most infamous).

There are several characteristics that a company, in order to define itself as truly innovative, must possess: to have a purpose, that is, the reason why the company exists beyond enriching investors; the ability to experiment, and therefore to quickly realize new ideas at a low price; collaboration between the company's sectors and those who are part of it; and the ability to transform simple concepts into attractive and easy-to-use products. In addition to all this, however, it must have the ability to *look beyond the present*, which of course includes all those activities that are habitually classified as open innovation.

It is clear that open innovation is an issue from which large companies, if they want to renew themselves successfully, cannot exempt themselves. Those who take this path often turn to young innovative companies, which in turn benefit from mingling with large ones, seizing opportunities for growth not only in a professional way, but also in a financial one. A virtuous circle that, given the growing importance of digital in medicine, can produce very interesting results, especially in the health sector. And the driving force behind health innovation are the startups. Digital innovation is transforming health from a simple state to a daily practice that indeed passes through digital tools and solutions. This paradigm shift in the concept of health allows startups to present themselves as real drivers of transformation, able to grasp the needs of the market and transform them into projects with a high innovative value. More and more often, pharmaceutical companies and companies in the entire health sector will be able to adopt models and approaches focused on the person, and startups represent, in a particular way, a new method for implementing that business strategy that is already revolutionizing the method of conceiving and practicing health.

Roberto's Vision

Open innovation means using processes that take place outside large companies. This method is particularly effective in the digital sector, where the risk of change is higher, precisely because of the speed at which it is triggered. Relying on innovative processes that take place outside large companies, allows, for those who develop projects, a greater degree of freedom and a greater predisposition to experimentation and creative thinking. Large organizations cannot afford to put so many projects in the pipeline and proceed through a long and complex trial-and-error process in order to achieve results. And yet, that's exactly how innovations are generated. This is where the value of startups comes into play. Unlike a large company, a startup lives on the innovative flows that it manages to generate. This gives it greater organizational flexibility so it can take on the risks related to verticalization in a specific production area. The large organization can take advantage of this opportunity by accelerating the development processes of the most promising startups and integrating them into their operational flows. It is a winning model, the only one through which it is possible to think of innovating the health-care sector. There are diverse applications of the open innovation model in the world of life sciences. Just think of the Roche HealthBuilders, Pfizer Healthcare Hub, Novartis BIOME, Bayer G4A, and Almirall Digital Garden initiatives, which are all aimed at making sure that traditional organizations can respond to the needs of patients and all the different stakeholders of the health world in an innovative way, thanks to the contributions of startups, researchers, experts, and insiders from around the world. The development of all these initiatives in support of startups and emerging companies is also favored by the constant increase in the investments made in digital health.

For investments, 2020 was a record year, with about $21.5 billion raised globally in every sector of the health-care innovation industry, as StartUp Health reports.[1] The global market of digital health is expected to generate revenue of $884.1 billion, proceeding to a compound annual growth rate (CAGR) of 21.8 percent between 2020 and 2030. This growth is driven by the ever-increasing demand for remote patient-monitoring services, the upsurge in the number of smartphone and tablet users, growing government support for digital health solutions, advances in mobile health-care applications, and an increased need for advanced health-care information systems.[2]

It is certainly not the only method by which innovation can be made, but targeted funding and operational support, on important initiatives, clearly help the development of these initiatives in an incontrovertible way. Many of these transformations are not coming from very large organizations, which are in fact very strong in their role, that is, involved in incremental research and therefore in improving something that is already known. But, as in all the other sectors that have been completely transformed, radical innovation comes precisely from startups, from the teams that are aware that they have about 90 percent chance of failure. It is precisely this strong evolutionary pressure that allows them to experiment in directions forbidden to large organizations that, as mentioned, are already centered on their business. And from the point of view of Digital Health, this movement now has over 20,000 companies in the world that are actually innovating from many different angles: trying to reinvent all aspects of the processes of care and education and trying to imagine how these can work. Today, it's probably easy to have ideas; the real challenge is making these ideas a reality. There is an unlimited number of ideas, and from this point of view, for those who propose themselves in this field, there is enormous space, especially in a local or even hyper-local dimension.

AlmirallShare and Digital Garden

The pharmaceutical multinational Almirall has launched two different initiatives: AlmirallShare and Digital Garden, both with the aim of identifying new resources for the treatment of dermatological diseases.

AlmirallShare was launched in 2017 with the aim of facilitating collaborations in dermatological research and accelerating the generation of new treatments for skin diseases, bringing together the science and creativity of experts from all over the world with the expertise of Almirall. Since then, more than 900 scientists have joined, and more than 400 proposals have been received.

In 2019, however, the Digital Garden accelerator was inaugurated to encourage and support the development of services and solutions that address current and future dermatological challenges. For the selected team, the program involves a 9-month acceleration path, financial support of up to 50,000 euros for the development of innovative products, and mentoring and partnership support activities. In addition, they have the possibility of implementing new technologies within the hospitals of Barcelona, which will serve as a test bed for pilot solutions.

Bayer G4A

Today the concept of health and well-being is experiencing a profound change, made possible by the implementation of new technologies and a paradigm shift in the conception of products and services that increasingly focus on people, animals, and plants.

Bayer G4A is an international program that supports innovative startups around the world operating in the life sciences sectors. The G4A network has its headquarters in Berlin, and houses the accelerator dedicated to digital health. It has now grown and has plans for dedicated programs in the cities of Barcelona, Shanghai, Tokyo, and Moscow. Other international headquarters are leaders in their cities with initiatives, events, and related activities.

The global G4A program, led by Bayer and active in 35 countries, is directed toward promising entrepreneurs whose goal is generating a significant impact in the health and assistance sectors through the implementation of digital technologies. G4A acts through the activation of business partnerships, funding, mentorship activities, and access to support networks, according to an approach based on the co-creation of innovative solutions. The program, initially called Grants4Apps, was launched in Berlin in 2013, with the original goal of funding smartphone applications. Over the years, the mission has expanded, embracing a wider spectrum of solutions and encompassing Venture Design, to conceive new products and revenues using the behavioral design scheme. To date, the G4A portfolio has more than 140 companies operating in the digital health field and the number is in a growth trend.

Frontiers Health

Designed as a spin-off event of Frontiers Conferences, producing international events about technology and innovation since 2005, over the last years Frontiers Health emerged as one of the premier conferences in the digital health space, combining a unique mix of attendees from life-science companies, health innovation hubs, insurance companies, investment funds, and startups. It provides a unique platform to discuss how innovations are transforming health care. The annual global event taking place in Berlin usually gathers around 600+ industry experts from 30 countries, who come together to discuss all aspects of digital health innovation, including digital therapies, breakthrough technologies, patient-centricity, health-care transformation, and so on. In light of the Covid-19 pandemic, Frontiers Health has been holding in a hybrid format, both offline and online, running dedicated local hubs from Italy, Germany, Finland, Spain, the United States, and more locations. Such format gives flexibility to attend the event from any location and get access to the top digital health community, ensuring Frontiers Health as a unique platform for deal making, networking, and learning. Of course, such a gathering of expertise has been committed to explore how digital health is being leveraged as a strategic pillar to the response of the pandemic, focusing on strategic topics such as digital therapeutics, health-care policies to foster innovation, insurtech, virtual clinical trials, artificial intelligence and virtual reality, investment strategies, and data science. In the midst of the first months of Covid-19's spread in 2020, Frontiers Health promptly launched the special initiative "Health Innovation Ecosystem Fighting Covid-19," a comprehensive map of the most active global players providing concrete solutions to mitigate the pandemic, with the aim to improve coordination and facilitate cooperation and scalability.[3]

Healthware Labs and Healthware Life Hub

Healthware Labs was founded in 2015 and soon established itself as one of the most advanced companies in innovation consulting for the life-sciences industry; it was also recognized by PM360 as one of the "Innovators 2015." Its strengths are the innovation of digital technology to support the pharmaceutical sector, the recognized leadership in the field of digital health, its many partnerships, and direct access to thousands of startups, all made available to new companies that seek to implement health innovation on a vast scale. Today, thanks to its having one of the largest networks of startups and agreements, Healthware Labs specializes in the co-development of projects dedicated to prevention, predictive health, and digital therapies. It is difficult, or too risky, for large companies to produce radical innovation with traditional systems, so much so that the processes of change and renewal almost never take place within them.

On the contrary, startups and investors are able to produce a continuous flow of innovation that creates new markets or disruptively modifies existing ones. And this indeed is the advantage offered by companies such as Healthware Labs. Any company that wants to convert to open innovation must connect to the startup ecosystem, and Healthware Labs, in this regard, represents a hub of excellence. That is because it provides companies with all the tools they require for introducing innovation methodologies within the existing business model, with a pool of consultants constantly experimenting with innovative trends, thinking about how to apply them in the field of health and how to develop them together with the company.

On the initiative of Healthware Labs, in 2021, the Healthware Life Hub Accelerator program was born. The program aims at offering startups a customized mentoring path to accelerate their growth and identify the best partners and ecosystems for new business opportunities. The headquarters of the Healthware Life Hub Accelerator is in Italy, in Salerno at the Palazzo Innovazione, a co-creation space focused on digital innovation housed in a former 11th-century monastery right in the region where the first school of medicine was born, a sort of ancestor of modern universities, as historically documented. There are places that are also sites of the work of the first female doctor, Trotula of Salerno.

HealthXL

HealthXL is a global community of experts that seeks to facilitate and promote the adoption of digital health solutions. Thanks to a data-driven collaborative platform that monitors over 50,000 health-care systems and academic centers, HealthXL's team is made up of industry experts, investors, data analysts, and health professionals. Working together, they produce reports and market and business analyses to identify new research, partnership, and investment opportunities in the digital health sector. HealthXL also organizes events and global gatherings on specific topics to discuss and continue to fuel the innovation of the digital health scene internationally. The events are a meeting point for community members who contribute in this way in the evolution of the health-care industry.

Johnson & Johnson Innovation Labs (JLABS)

JLABS represents a network of incubators operating in the field of life sciences that aims at accelerating innovative solutions in the pharmaceutical, diagnostic, and health-tech sectors, to improve the health and well-being of patients all over the world.

The labs seek to pursue these objectives by creating optimal environments for young companies to be able to grow and refine their research and development activities, promoting connections with large companies and starting entrepreneurial training programs—without affecting the intellectual property that underlies innovation. There are about 8 labs located in North America, Europe, and the Far East, plus other affiliated centers globally.

Novartis Biome

The Novartis Biome is a digital innovation lab powered by Novartis. It aims to empower and engender health-tech companies and people passionate about disrupting health-care through the use of data and digital technologies. This initiative allows teams to co-develop digital solutions alongside specific therapeutic offerings, research activities, and business processes within Novartis. At the same time, Biome provides external innovators with the resources and opportunities to validate their solutions through access to regulatory, medical, or legal expertise; clinical trial design; market access; and, in some cases, investment and financing. the Novartis Biome is a growing network of innovation hubs, some already in place (e.g., United Kingdom, France, India, and United States), and others about to launch (e.g., Spain, Canada, and Germany) with plans of further expansion across three continents.

Open Accelerator

Open Accelerator is the international acceleration program for start-ups in life sciences, created by Zcube—Zambon Research Venture—for identifying and financing the best solutions that will define the future of health. Created in 2016, Open Accelerator has grown over the years, extending its scope and calls to tender internationally since its second edition. The aim of the program is identifying projects and startups that create transformative experiences for the patient throughout his or her healing process, from healthy living to awareness and commitment, to prevention, diagnosis, disease management, and the follow-up phase.

Patients' Digital Health Awards

The Patients' Digital Health Awards (PDHA) is promoted by the Digital Health Academy in collaboration with 50 patient associations and the unconditional contribution of the MSD Foundation. The PDHA initiative was conceived to consider digital health ideas and projects from the patient perspective.

During the PDHA evaluation process, patients are the ones to give feedback and evaluate the projects. The Awards Committee is composed of 50 patient associations together with digital health experts.

This model is a marked divergence from other similar competitions, where entries are usually assessed by health-care experts or professionals only. It also means that the contestants get an opportunity to interact with the patients directly and follow the patients' user path when they are getting treatment. This setup helps to achieve the overall goal of making digital health solutions more human and patient-centric. The awards have been running since 2018, and the 2020 edition has been adjusted to the post-pandemic reality, with the aim of giving additional visibility to Covid-related digital health solutions for the benefit of the whole health-care ecosystem.

Pfizer Healthcare Hubs

The hubs network created by Pfizer aims at working on digital solutions for the patient, addressing itself not only to startups, but also to spin-offs, tech companies, and other types of innovators. A type of personalized support is provided, which, based on specific needs, can include services such as access to the network of internal experts, support activities, market analysis, and support to the sales and partnership strategies. To date, there are 15 hubs internationally through which Pfizer accelerates the placing on the market of innovative products that guarantee a better level of care for the patient.

Roche HealthBuilders

HealthBuilders represents the first open innovation program dedicated to health conceived and realized by the Italian branch of the Swiss multinational Roche. The initiative selects breakthrough ideas for maximizing the potential of digital technologies in the health process. In particular, Roche aims at intercepting cutting-edge solutions in terms of the economic and social sustainability of the healthcare system and of the customer experience of the patient, his or her caregiver, and all stakeholders in the therapeutic areas of oncology, rare diseases, and neuroscience. In these areas, Roche evaluates innovative solutions that include digital devices, apps, remote monitoring systems, social networks, wearables, and virtual/augmented reality technologies, as well as instant messaging, voice over internet protocol (VoIP), the internet of things, big data, and AI.

StartUp Health

StartUp Health is an organization founded in 2011 to support digital health-care companies and help them during their growth. It is based in New York and has organized numerous meetings between entrepreneurs and potential investors to discuss the challenges and opportunities that are on the horizon. Spread over 26 countries and six continents, StartUp Health is organizing and investing in a global army of health transformers and has the largest portfolio of companies operating in digital health worldwide. The goal for the next 25 years is very ambitious: improving the well-being of all the inhabitants of the planet. To succeed, it has created a worldwide network of over 200,000 actors among innovators, industry leaders, and investors committed to supporting entrepreneurs in their effort to reinvent health and well-being.

In recent years, StartUp Health has benefited from new investments, including a particularly substantial one ($31 million) from Novartis, Ping An Group, Chiesi Group, GuideWell, Otsuka, Masimo, and other private investors.

"From day one, we had a vision synchronized with the leadership of Novartis, Ping An Group, Chiesi Group, GuideWell, Otsuka, and our partner community," said Steven Krein, co-founder and CEO of StartUp Health. "We believe that it is necessary to have unique collaborations between the entrepreneurs driving innovation and world leaders in the industry in order to solve today's most complex healthcare challenges."

For Unity Stoakes, co-founder and president of StartUp Health, every aspect of health care is undergoing a profound process of renewal, and the best way to speed it up is to refine collaboration across the various stakeholders, providing both entrepreneurs and innovators with support, skills, and resources to grow their business.

StartUp Health is carrying out a long-term mission (25 years) called Moonshot. "For us, Moonshot is a powerful metaphor for addressing the health challenges of our time. If we can put a man on the moon, then we know that we can also transform global health, curing diseases and providing care to all people, regardless of location or income." Guided by this definition and vision, Startup Health has gathered in their portfolio more than 230 companies, from six continents and 20 countries, divided into 10 Health Moonshots (Access to Care, Cost to Zero, Cure Disease, End to Cancer, Women's Health, Children's Health, Nutrition and Fitness, Brain Health, Happiness and Mental Health, and Longevity).

Vertical

Vertical is a Helsinki-based consulting group specializing in the creation of open innovation processes, the management of accelerators and incubators, and the development of innovation programs tailored to companies.

Born as an accelerator, today Vertical helps startups from all over the world to grow strategically and forge partnerships with diverse stakeholders in the sector. At Vertical, a team of experts offers startups three different types of services divided as follows:

- Collaboration for rapidly developing technology or business models by discussion with other startups, companies, or end users
- Strategy for identifying and designing new business opportunities
- Operation for finding the right strategic partners interested in investing or entering into agreements

Vertical's services thus enable emerging startups to grow by strengthening their business model based on the real needs of the market and at the same time, entering into discussion with market leaders such as Samsung, with food industry players such as Fazer, and major healthcare providers, including the Hospital District of Helsinki and Uusimaa (HUS).

Guest Perspectives

UNITY STOAKES
Co-founder and President, Startup Health

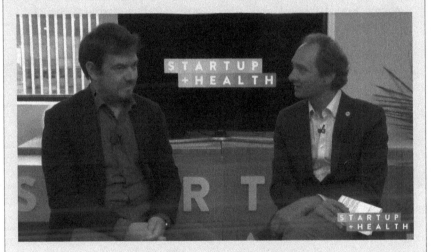

Roberto Ascione and Unity Stoakes

Credit: Roberto Ascione – private archives

At StartUp Health, we believe that anything is possible with the right mindset and entrepreneurial spirit. We also know that when we bring together people united by the same passion to improve everyone's lives and push them to achieve a common goal, something magical happens.

We live in a unique moment in the history of health care, where solutions coexist that, if properly coordinated, could improve access to care (at ever-decreasing costs) for billions of people. What's needed now is to work together as a single ecosystem and collaboratively support those with an innovative mindset in the field of healthcare.

Artificial intelligence, blockchain, data, virtual reality, mobile connectivity, advanced predictive analytics solutions, and new business models are

(Continues)

(Continued)

changing healthcare, and this is creating an unprecedented wave of innovation. For the past decade we have been building a global health moonshot factory to help a new generation of innovators solve the world's biggest health challenges like ending cancer and curing disease, pandemic response, mental health and brain health and longevity. Through a collaborative innovation platform, we are able to speed up innovation and accelerate impact.

We monitor huge amounts of information and data about where the money is flowing, what business models are working, who's investing in what subsectors and regions, and how companies can access them. When we began our company, there was little capital flowing and virtually no ecosystem to support early-stage health innovation. Not only has that changed, but in a post-pandemic world the entire landscape has shifted and transformed overnight.

In March 2020, we instantly recalibrated to put in motion a global plan to speed up the progress being made. We have launched a new subscription model to make it easier for investors to back health moonshots and to provide funding to hundreds and one day thousands of companies that will each revamp a different aspect of the system and, together, become what transforms the entire industry.

It's exciting to see how the global ecosystem continues to evolve and grow. We are more optimistic than ever that entrepreneurs and innovators—Health Transformers—have the potential to improve the health and well-being of everyone in the world in the next 25 years.

TANJA DOWE
CEO, Debiopharm

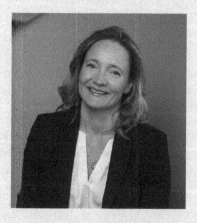

Tanja Dowe
Credit: Tania Dowe – private archives

Innovations Will Take Place in a Sharing Ecosystem

Pharma's frame of reference is changing. The shift is coming from outside pharma, from the pressing need to reduce health-care costs, and it is facilitated by leaps in data, AI, and digital tools. There are two main tangents of change.

First, our main customer persona is changing quickly from health-care provider to patient (or health consumer), and that consumer comes with the attitude of a digital native teenager. They will not accept the level of information and services that past generations have accepted.

Second, the digital-native generation is also turning our society into a sharing economy—crowdsourcing, open source, recycling, you name it, are the norm for them. In the sharing economy, consumers are also ready to share their health data to benefit others and in return expect benefits to themselves. There will be larger and more versatile data aggregates available as raw material for innovations.

So here you have an involved health consumer and data like you never had before. How does pharma innovate in this ecosystem? Not like before, with a handful of start-ups in an endless *pilotitis*. You have to become a committed part of this ecosystem and co-create the future with the other ecosystem players. And you also have to lose sight of the barriers for change, so that the focus does not remain in how to overcome today's obstacles. It is futile to think about them, because in a real seismic change of an industry the problems and barriers will not remain the same.

Strategic Investments to Build Platforms

We asked ourselves the question, what can the strategic investment fund of a pharma company do to promote this ecosystem thinking? Our decision was to invest in digital health start-ups that will challenge pharma thinking from two perspectives: how we develop drugs, and how we treat patients (in our case, we focus on oncology patients).

So far we have invested in eight start-ups that approach these two questions from different angles, creating mini-ecosystems. BC Platforms, Novadiscovery, Nucleai, and Carevive are changing the way we see drug development, and Voluntis, Oncomfort, and Kaiku Health (now exited) help us find ways to treat patients beyond drugs. Our aim is to create collaboration opportunities for them with our pharmaceutical development colleagues at Debiopharm, but also with each other and with other ecosystem players.

Our job is not done. We will continue investing in new entrants to these ecosystems. Our dream is that with time, these ecosystems will turn into highly successful platforms for the future of health.

(Continues)

(*Continued*)

KRISTIN MILBURN
Managing Director, Healthware Labs

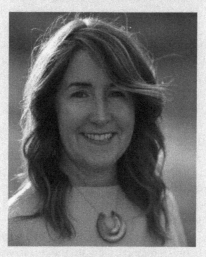

Kristin Milburn
Credits: Frontiers Health

Healthware Labs was founded at a time when we knew healthcare was undergoing a massive amount of change due to the acceleration of technological advances and the resulting digital transformation. The term "digital health" was just beginning to become part of the regular lexicon in the health-care space and our clients were looking for guidance to better understand what was happening and how to approach digital health in their own businesses.

One method we use to help our clients develop innovative digital health solutions is called *design thinking*. Design thinking is a human-centered methodology used to find creative solutions to real-world problems. The first step in this process is the most critical and that is to *empathize* with your target audience. In the world of healthcare that means truly understanding the lived experience of the patient's life, outside the doctor's office, with whatever condition they are facing. Let's take migraines, for example, how does someone adapt their life when they feel a migraine coming on? When you truly put yourself in the shoes of someone else, you can better imagine ways to leverage technology to build a solution to help meet their needs. The next step is to accurately *define* the problem, or as we call them "opportunity spaces"—areas that could benefit from a new solution. Step three is the fun part and that is to *ideate* or brainstorm for potential solutions, pulling ideas from other industries and applying them to this challenge.

Many times we'll find that there are start-ups already addressing a particular challenge. This is no surprise, as many successful start-ups are founded based on unmet needs of patients or a challenge—they watched a family member or friend endure when confronted with a disease or newly diagnosed condition. So before proceeding to build a new solution from scratch we'll run a "search and vet" or an open innovation challenge to get the word out that we're seeking solutions for our client and help them sort through various submissions that can potentially best meet their needs. When we find a start-up that matches the needs identified we'll partner with the winning solution and *co-create* a customized program that makes the most sense. In doing so, we are typically bringing together a large Fortune 100 company with over 100,000 employees worldwide and a small start-up with sometimes less than 50 people, which can make for a tricky partnership. It's important to remember that both sides come to the table with strengths; start-ups have agility and speed and the ability to pivot to adapt to needs quickly. Pharmaceutical companies have deep expertise in the therapeutic areas they cover and vast resources in areas such as market access and commercialization. While these partnerships may not be done easily or quickly, if managed appropriately it can be a win-win-win: a win-win for the two companies involved and, more importantly, a win for the patients for which they are building a solution. As long as the patient's needs remain front and center throughout the process, we've found these partnerships can be quite successful. And that brings us to the fifth and final step of the design thinking process and that is to *test* the solution in the real world with real patients.

It's extremely gratifying to know that, after all the hard work getting your solution into the hands of patients, you can make a meaningful impact on their day-to-day lives and this is what motivates me and everyone at Healthware Labs to do what we do.

(*Continues*)

(Continued)

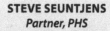

STEVE SEUNTJENS
Partner, PHS

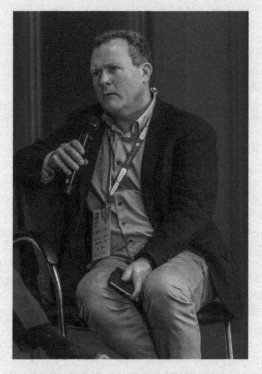

Steve Seuntjens at Frontiers Health
Credit: Steve Seuntjens, Partner, PHS.

For the last 15 years, my focus has been on supporting and investing in individual-centric, scienced-backed, digitally enabled health solutions. During this period, we have seen a convergence, allowing individuals to become active participants in their health versus passive recipients.

Today there are hundreds of thousands of applications for individuals and health professionals providing a point of access and vital information toward support of care. We see wearables going beyond an individual well-being tool toward being prescribed to manage a chronic condition. The promise of digital solutions is beginning to show its strength toward offering real-time access as well as reliability and affordability. Today's solutions offload some of the burden of care on overstretched health systems by providing preventative measures, triaging of individuals, and remote monitoring. Investment in the digital health space has grown from $1 billion annually to over 20 times this in the last 10 years.

An illustration of a few solutions may provide a more tangible understanding on the health transformation underway; SkinVision and Pacifica, now Sanvello, are two solution examples I have been involved with from my role as an investor.

SkinVision allows for individual awareness and early detection of the most common types of skin cancer. It is a mobile application, providing awareness on prevention elements as well as deeper information surrounding the types and risks of skin cancer. Through a smartphone photo (automatically taken with no additional attachments) a clinically validated risk assessment is provided within 30 seconds through AI/ML technology, providing a low-risk or high-risk reading. The solution has found over 90,000 skin cancer lesions and is utilized by millions.

Skin cancer is the most common type of cancer with an increasing incidence. Early detection significantly reduces complications and enhances life. There is a shortage of specialists and wait times are increasing. SkinVision's mission is to save 250,000 lives in the next decade by supporting individuals to get to the right doctor at the right time. Understanding the risk of a particular lesion allows for the appropriate action to be taken. This supports to reduce wait times and provides better outcomes for those with the most urgent needs.

Sanvello offers clinically proven mental health therapies for individuals in the areas of stress, anxiety, and depression. It is a mobile application, meeting individuals where they are in moments of need and surrounding them with tools and strategies that provide effective relief.

The pandemic has highlighted the growing need for access and support in this area. Only one in three of those suffering from mental health is known to the health system. An overstretched health system and lack of professionals cannot singularly deal with a crisis of this magnitude. Access to proven and reliable solutions such as Sanvello supports in meeting individual health needs while reducing the burden on the health system.

Sanvello is now part of United Health Group and is serving millions of individuals in need of mental health support.

(*Continues*)

(Continued)

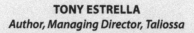

TONY ESTRELLA
Author, Managing Director, Taliossa

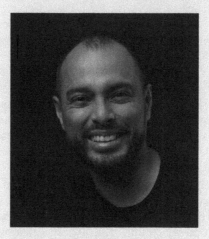

Tony Estrella
Credit: Tony Estrella

In recent years, several leading health-care companies have embraced the model of open innovation. By pulling back the curtains of secrecy, leading organizations are instead embracing a model of transparency with external partners, increasing the likelihood for successfully solving complex business challenges.

Why? Every organization has its own core strengths or capabilities. But this also means a company has blind spots. And broadly speaking in health care, these weaknesses include knowing how to change consumer behavior, iterating rapidly for technology-led solutions—both hardware and software—and leveraging all forms of data effectively.

Outside of health care, the promise for such work is clear. Platforms like Quirky bring together people for co-creation and collaboration. Technology companies like Samsung have embraced an open innovation model for years—with significant business impact—through its group in Silicon Valley. And example solutions abound, including a Domino's Pizza working with Nuro to offer autonomous pizza delivery in the United States.

It is truly refreshing to see a growing number of examples within health care, such as Bayer's G4A program for digital health startups and GSK's DPAc co-creation program with academia. These programs illustrate what is necessary to truly embrace open innovation. Identify core challenges. Figure out and accept your blind spots. And then reach out to a community with the mindset of "How can we solve problems together?"

As an entrepreneur, innovation executive, podcaster, and author, I'm an active leader in driving my own version of open innovation in Asia Pacific. I first lead by tapping into the power of storytelling. Similar to the influence *Star Trek* had on the aspirations of space travel and subsequent growth of the industry, my podcasts and writing—both fiction and non-fiction—aim to provide a roadmap to the future of open innovation in health care. Through my work with FutureProofing Healthcare, a group supported by Roche, we leverage various media including podcasts to create a shared vision.

In parallel, through my company Taliossa, I help create ecosystems to solve complex business challenges to achieve this shared vision of health care. This includes going outside of traditional stakeholders and finding creative ways to include other industries such as insurance, banking, and consumer technology organizations. We guide these programs through our proven methodology which first establishes joint problem statements across the ecosystem, and then emphasizes using data to make quick adjustments in deploying solutions at various levels of scale.

One example customer journey we are actively reinventing is helping people with limited incomes tap into innovative fintech solutions to help afford personalized health-care solutions in cancer. In other words, we are striving to eliminate the affordability gap.

Through continued open innovation programs, the future is bright for improving the health outcomes for individuals around the world.

Notes

1. StartUp Health. "Record-breaking year for health innovation funding sets the stage for new era of health moonshot progress," HealthTransformer.co, January 6, 2021. Available at: https://healthtransformer.co/record-breaking-year-for-health-innovation-funding-sets-the-stage-for-new-era-of-health-moonshot-fe0bd379a715.
2. ResearchAndMarkets.com. "Global digital health markets 2020–2030: Increasing number of partnerships and agreements & rising

number of acquisitions," press release, November 18, 2020. Available at: https://www.prnewswire.com/news-releases/global-digital-health-markets-2020-2030-increasing-number-of-partnerships-and-agreements-rising-number-of-acquisitions-301175892.html.

3. Frontiers in Health. "Health innovation ecosystem fighting Covid-19," Frontiers.Health, 2020. Available at: https://www.frontiers.health/download-fh-map/.

CHAPTER 9

Lifestyle as Medicine

From Self-Empowerment to Lifestyle as Medicine

There is nothing new about the idea that diet, exercise, and other lifestyle factors affect our health and well-being. What is new instead is being able to take advantage of digital technologies to encourage us in these activities for improving our health. There is much talk about empowerment, on a personal level (i.e., self-empowerment), referring precisely to all those measures that the individual can implement in order to feel more responsible, more at the center of his or her own life, and in a better state of health. In traditional therapies, empowerment is used for addressing issues related to clinical interventions of chronic diseases, for the prevention and promotion of good health as well as to treat stress or better manage a disability. The advent of digital technologies has allowed these techniques to be extended to a wider audience, where many of the practices in use can be coded within a program or app and used through a smartphone. Techniques that trace their origins back millennia, such as yoga, can now be made available through a digital system that can guide the user toward states of relaxation and meditation. The effects that music has always had on human physiology and psychology can now come through new technologies, with algorithms able to process vast musical libraries from which to extract sequences of songs capable of generating, in those who listen to them, a general improvement in their mood and other physiological aspects related to it, such as tachycardia or breathing frequency. In this scenario, there is a growing importance of *health coaches*, that is, all those digital programs that help one to adopt a healthier lifestyle, lose weight, or sleep better. The health coach market is a booming one, bearing in mind that in 2019 about 121,000 health coaches were available in the United States. In an increasingly broad sense, we can therefore speak of *lifestyle as medicine* to refer to all those processes that lead to a general improvement in the health of the individual. An example of such solutions can be Sleepio, a digital program that helps improve the quality of sleep, which we will also talk about later.

Roberto's Vision

Many pathologies are determined by biological aspects and, more specifically, by a person's genetic makeup. But many others are entirely or largely defined by other factors such as nutrition, a sedentary lifestyle, or a bad lifestyle in general. If this is true, it is clear that a number of effective interventions on these aspects can have extremely beneficial effects on the health of each one of us. To be totally frank, operations in this field are not a novelty in the strict sense, nor do they come about as a consequence of entering the digital age: for example, for many years, diabetes campaigns have focused on messages that promote greater physical activity, the adoption of a healthier and more balanced eating style, and so on. But the advent of digital has nevertheless introduced a breath of fresh air into this field. Today, digital tools make it possible to have a wealth of information quickly accessible and various smartphone apps make it possible to access a range of services that let one have a whole series of behavioral advice in an intelligent, pleasant, and rapid way. Not only that, the advice, thanks to these new technologies, is given at the right time and in a way that is not only useful, but also pleasant for those who receive it. Precisely for this reason they are not perceived as medical interventions.

Consider for a moment the difficulty of absorbing the key points of a newspaper article or a magazine, which is simply to be read. Apps and other digital technologies are useful and persuasive precisely because they arrive contextualized with respect to everyday activities. They are also pleasant from the point of view of design and engaging (i.e., actually interesting to use). The advent of digital, therefore, has made these behavioral suggestions enormously more effective and measurable than in the recent past, effectively making them useful remedies. I like to call this approach "lifestyle as medicine" since user-centric digital solutions that are noninvasive, useful, and intelligent, and pleasant in design, encourage us to adopt behaviors that are beneficial for our health and well-being in general. Consider, for example, the importance of receiving dietary advice calibrated on what one's own preferences are. There will be no suggestions regarding unwelcome foods or flavors! In addition, the tips will arrive at the right time of day, when you are thinking about what to cook for dinner and are shopping, instead of close to meal-time, which would make the suggestion useless. An app that realizes that we are in the supermarket and therefore directs us toward a certain type of food can help us make a more conscious and useful purchase. Maybe it recognizes the packaging of the product we are going to buy or instead advises us of a certain type of nutrient mix rather than another, because it knows our diet and our tastes, and helps us to stock our pantry in the best way for us. The ease of use, design, and accuracy of the information contained in these applica-tions, the help deriving from geolocation or food recognition, will make it easier and more concretely feasible to adopt a correct life-style. Consequently, it will be more pleasant to carry out actions that will lead to a general improvement in the state of health.

This same type of approach is applicable to many other areas. For example, it has been studied that a certain type of music and certain types of sounds have a beneficial effect on concentration and relaxation as well as decreasing the general stress levels of those who listen to them. There are apps that, thanks to sophisticated algo-rithms that are constantly being refined, are able to understand what kind of sound or music can benefit an individual in relation to a series of issues such as stress, anxiety, insomnia, or concentration. The algorithms of these applications record signals such as breathing frequency or heartbeat and develop, in response, a music playlist that can induce relaxation, and in general stimulate a positive response of the organism. This type of therapy is, of course, being rigorously scientifically verified, but it is clear that a solution that is able to pro-vide a certain type of music that leads to a reduction in stress will certainly have positive effects, for example, from a cardiovascular point of view. Starting from this assumption, who knows whether or not we can activate, through apps of this type, those mechanisms that the human organism is very well equipped to reduce, for exam-ple, blood pressure, which we know is a very important risk factor for cardiovascular diseases. Yoga, music, and relaxation techniques are all practices that have existed before the advent of digital and that for hundreds of years have been recognized as able to provide well-being, on an emotional and physical level: they are nothing more than strategies for activating the skills inherent in our body. Digital technologies draw on the same practices used for millennia, making them accessible to a vast quantity of people, improving the relationship with their bodies, and ultimately improving their health.

Headspace

Headspace is a digital service that offers guided meditation sessions and mindfulness training directly through the web or through apps. Headspace was founded in May 2010 by Andy Puddicombe (a former Buddhist monk) and Rich Pierson (an expert in marketing and new brand development). The story of its conception is quite interesting and deserves to be told. It all began in 1994 when Puddicombe interrupted his university studies in sports sciences and, at the age of 22, went to Asia to become a Buddhist monk. There, he spent 10 years on pilgrimages between Nepal, India, Burma, Thailand, Australia, and Russia, always looking for a deep and satisfying meditative technique. In 2004 he returned to England with a mission: to make meditation accessible, relevant, and beneficial to as many people as possible.

He opened a meditation clinic in London, and this is where he met his future business partner, Rich Pierson. "Rich had all these creative skills," says Puddicombe, "and I had the necessary experience given by my past as a monk. We combined the two to create something that could make meditation truly within everyone's reach." Initially, Headspace was established as an event company that organized awareness meetings in and around London. But the continuous request from participants to have a tool to use these techniques outside of the meetings in everyday life led Puddicombe and Pierson to study the development of a mobile app. The first version of the Headspace app was launched in 2012, and more than 50 employees are currently working on the project. The staff is divided between the locations of Santa Monica and San Francisco in California and London. The techniques used in the Headspace app have been refined and developed over many centuries. Their purpose is to cultivate awareness and compassion so that we can better understand both our mind and the world that surrounds us. In 2018, Headspace said it had over a million monthly users. Puddicombe and Pierson's app has also been used in a number of clinical trials, such as the one conducted by researchers at UCL (University College of London), funded by the British Heart Foundation, which examined the impact of workplace stress awareness in two large multinationals. The study found several significant benefits that Headspace use had on workers: increased well-being, reduced states of anxiety and depressive symptoms, reduction in diastolic blood pressure, an increase in perceived work control, and reduction of sleep-related problems.

HealthTunes

HealthTunes is a California company founded in 2016 by Walter Werzowa, musician, composer, and music producer. It is an audio-streaming service designed to improve the physical and mental health of those who use it. Depending on the patient's condition, Health-Tunes offers specific health and musical therapies. Doctors who collaborate with HealthTunes, in fact, create an actual therapeutic plan, *prescribing* the type of music (i.e., the *MusicMedicine*) that the patient will have to listen to, the quantity, and the length of time he or she will have to do it.

Doctors make personalized music playlists (the *therapies*), based on the diagnosis, symptoms, and syndromes of the patient. Music-Medicine works on three levels. First, it activates the emotional state of the patient, trying to improve it instantly. Second, it helps to recall the sensory memory. Finally, it acts physiologically, bringing back balance in the parasympathetic nervous system. For example, with playlists created for persons affected by Alzheimer's disease, it is possible to stimulate the production of dopamine, and a process of brain plasticity is activated that helps to regrow their neural connections. With playlists created for people with Parkinson's, in addition to the stimulation of dopamine, the music also stimulates a mechanism that leads the patients to having a more secure gait. Binaural tones (or binaural beats) are also used in the music of the various playlists. These are beats perceived by the brain when two sounds with a frequency of less than 1,500 Hz and with a difference of less than 30 Hz are heard separately through the earbuds. These beats are generated directly in the brain, according to a phenomenon identified and described as early as 1839 by Heinrich Wilhelm Dove. Experimental data have shown the effectiveness of the use of binaural beats in treatments against chronic pain, insomnia, anxiety, and heart rate.

Noom

"Helping people adopt a healthier lifestyle through changing their habits" is the mission of Noom, a company founded in 2008 by Saeju Jeong and Artem Petakov. Since 2016, Noom has launched an app to manage weight loss. Today the Noom app is used by over 50 million users who, after setting their weight-loss goal, can interact with and ask for support from over 1,300 coaches. Users can monitor not only their weight, but also their physical activity, blood pressure, and blood sugar. In addition, Noom also provides a food and diet database that includes 3.7 million articles. It is estimated that 64 percent of users have lost 5 percent or more of their body weight, thus greatly reducing the risk of diabetes and other diseases. The company is constantly expanding and in 2019 partnered with Eversana on a program to improve adherence to the therapy. Also in this direction is the partnership with Novo Nordisk for the realization of a training and psychological support program for patients taking pharmaceuticals for weight loss.

Sleepio

Sleepio is a digital program for sleep improvement with cognitive behavioral therapy techniques developed by sleep scientist Colin Espie together with the former insomnia sufferer Peter Hames. Developed by the company Big Health and used by over 12 million people, Sleepio provides a digital tool accessible via app and web for improving the quality of sleep. In June 2019, CVS Health, the largest U.S. drug reimbursement manager, began including Sleepio's app among the reimbursable drugs for tens of millions of people. Sleepio is used more like a video game for a single player, in which the user is looking for a better sleep, than as a clinical health program. Thanks to a virtual sleep expert, a user can learn cognitive techniques to help have or restore more natural patterns of sleep. Peter Hames, the chief executive of Big Health, said he had an idea for Sleepio after having suffered from insomnia. Hames taught himself to change his bad sleep habits, reading self-help books on cognitive behavioral therapy, especially those by Espie, a professor of sleep medicine at Oxford University. Successively, with Espie, he then founded Big Health to digitize the techniques.

Pioppi Protocol

Pioppi Protocol is an app that provides a guide on the lifestyle of the Mediterranean Diet, a nutritional model born in the small fishing village of Pioppi in the Cilento area of southern Italy. It has been scientifically proven that the inhabitants of Pioppi and of the Cilento live 10 years longer than their counterparts in other areas of the world, thanks not only to a healthier diet, but also to a healthier overall lifestyle. The Pioppi Protocol app, developed on the basis of the documentary *The Big Fat Fix*, by cardiologist Aseem Malhotra and filmmaker Donal O'Neill, makes the principles underlying the Mediterranean Diet lifestyle accessible digitally and one can learn, thanks to a virtual assistant, how to adopt a rhythm of life that has a healthier impact on our body and mind.

YourCoach.health

YourCoach.health is a solution that allows health coaches to guide those under their care holistically, creating a personalized path to improve or recover mental, physical, and emotional well-being. This solution was developed by Marina Borukhovich, an entrepreneur who turned her battle against cancer into a mission to customize health care. During her treatment journey, Marina understood the importance of healing emotionally and mentally in order to be truly well. She began to follow a specific diet, to practice boxing, and to look for health coaches who could support her, then she decided to become a health coach herself. This experience led Marina to found YourCoach to allow everyone to find the right health coach and, at the same time, facilitate the work of health coaches in following their patients.

Guest Perspective

WALTER WERZOWA
CEO, HealthTunes

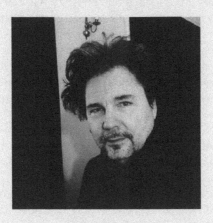

Walter Werzova
Credit: Evelyne Werzowa

Austrian-born Walter Werzowa is well known in the international music composing scene. With numerous television themes and movie scores to his credit, including films by Steven Spielberg and Wim Wenders, his most famous work is a sound that is instantly recognizable worldwide: Intel's audio branding jingle. In 2016, he founded HealthTunes, a streaming audio service that combines music with binaural beats and isochronic tones to improve physical and mental health based on a patient's condition.

"There is a new modality among us that is gradually transforming from a disruptive teenager to the wise and scientific professor, by the name 'MusicMedicine.' Initially doubted as acupuncture was in 1970s Western medicine's perception, MusicMedicine is increasingly gaining the interest of the health industry, and more importantly, winning the hearts, and especially the ears of patients.

"MusicMedicine not only shines in treatments for Alzheimer's, Parkinson's, chronic pain, insomnia, neonatal intensive care, ontology, and others, but it also is sought after by caregivers. We support the health of physicians and caregivers along with their patients.

(Continues)

(Continued)

"Better patient care also comes through the better well-being of the players. We placed innovative ideas, like MusicMedicine, in hospital recreation places, gardens, and anxiety-generating hospital machinery.

"Music foremost stimulates our mind and emotion, and it furthers collaboration and teamwork. Medical studies show MusicMedicine's physiological and cognitive benefits. Music not only makes us move, but it is also the force within that creates and recalls emotion. We collaborated with the department of medicine at the University of Vienna and the Vienna Philharmonic, and observed how human physiology is transformed with music. Listeners train breathing, heart rate, and heart rate variability to the music. When we add binaural beats (HealthTunes' proprietary therapy engine), we can focus on specific brain-wave entrainment.

"Our curated music streams positively stimulate the vagus nerve and with that, our parasympathetic nervous system.

"MusicMedicine is prescribed following precise therapeutic plans, and its effects are positively impacting patients and their close family members, care staff, and medical teams. This is one reason why two medical departments at the the University of California have validated and approved HealthTunes as music therapy.

"HealthTunes is spearheading a study at AKH-Vienna General Hospital to demonstrate the self-empowering effects of music. The study investigates the impact of sensory deprivation on patients after bone marrow transplantation surgery. The first results clearly show that when patients are allowed to choose the audio stimuli that best suit them, their physiology improves, leading to faster recovery.

"In combination with virtual reality, HealthTunes became a partner in multiple health projects."

PART II

Human Reflections

We are in the first months of 2021 and, among the consequences of the pandemic, we can observe an unprecedented acceleration to the digitization of medicine. A true leap of 10 years of digital evolution in a phenomenally short time. (In one of my interviews after the first period of the pandemic, I indeed said, "Ten years in ten days.") In fact, the pandemic has accelerated the large-scale spread and adoption of digital health solutions and tools such as sensors, health apps, wearable devices for continuous monitoring of biometric parameters, virtual assistants equipped with artificial intelligence (AI) that facilitate the doctor-patient relationship, digital platforms and services for remote medical care, and algorithms that generate physiological and behavioral digital biomarkers.

Why has this happened so broadly and so quickly? In other words, why did the adoption of these innovations literally explode? And again, is all of it destined to stay?

We start from the assumption that radical innovation on a large scale only happens when people have an actual unsatisfied need that innovation helps with or satisfies. When that happens, things have changed forever; there is no turning back. It is like jumping to a different level and after a while, you wonder how you ever used to do things the old way!

131

Let's look at it in greater detail. Although digital technologies have been part of our daily lives for several years, with the Covid-19 emergency a series of needs emerged with great force, needs that digital solutions had already resolved in other fields. With treatments being suspended during lockdown and distancing rules showing the limitations of traditional health care, there was the need for skills and services that could also be accessed remotely. The absolute need to integrate traditional medicine with digital medicine has become even more evident, as has the crucial role of digital health in offering new communication dynamics between doctor and patient. The scarcity or impossibility of physical access to doctors and hospitals was therefore the first driver that gave impetus to the adoption of telemedicine, widespread, in any case, for over 20 years. The difficulty of finding drugs and going to pharmacies has instead fostered the growth of home delivery and digital pharmacy services in general. The strong pressure on hospital facilities due to the management of the Covid-19 patients and the objective risk of contagion has pushed toward the adoption of remote monitoring of chronic diseases and the development of digital therapies.

Even the bodies responsible for regulating the placing on the market of drugs and devices, such as the U.S. Federal Drug Administration (FDA), also quickly adjusted their policies so as to allow the use of tools (that had proven their safety) as emergency measures, but it was later evident that this approach could be made stable to allow these tools to respond to the needs of patients and doctors as quickly as possible in any type of situation.

It is now clear that health management in the future will be based on the digitization of the entire healthcare process, with innovative solutions being developed increasingly around the health needs of people that hopefully will also guide the choices of decision-makers and health-care systems.

In the near future, the approach to health will be increasingly preventive and less reactive, personalized for each individual, based on billions of processed datapoints, predictive of the main risks and pathologies, and integrated on several levels of care. The culture of health-care data will be increasingly important—not only for the mere control and monitoring of the patient—but above all as a tool of a preventive diagnostic nature and contributing to large-scale health-care planning.

This pandemic has made it clear, once again, that there can be no economy, no society, without good health. And it is evident, now more than ever, why digital is a strategic tool that facilitates and, in many cases, allows the doctor-patient relationship to exist, thus ensuring the continuity of access to care not only for Covid-19 patients, to keep with the pandemic example, but also for those with other pathologies whose treatments are currently disrupted and for which there is a need to rethink the future of medicine and health management.

CHAPTER 10

The New Physicians and Patients

Empowered Doctors
and Health Consumers

An Ever-Increasing Pressure

In this 21st century, the advent of the internet alone has changed the relationship between the doctor and the patient. The vast amount of information, images, and videos invaded our lives and changed the way we behave, influencing as never before the construction of people's thinking and even determining their actions. Examples of all this are before our eyes, and all of us are affected by it.

Humanity has never had so much information and knowledge available; it's just a mouse-click away. All this, however, though it has undoubtedly changed history, has not brought us to an era of true widespread knowledge. On the contrary, it almost seems that too much information, along with too many stimuli, are causing a problem of attention and undermining the ability to dig deeper. As Stan Lee, the last true modern philosopher, had Spider-Man say, "With great power comes great responsibility." And so, it would take a great effort of culture on the part of each of us to make the most of the opportunity of so much knowledge that the web makes available to us. A great cultural effort is required in order to judge and select the sources of origin of a given data, to understand what is important, and to discard what is not. This reasoning is complex and takes us away from the objectives of our reflection.

Let us consider the part more directly related to the theme of health. Never before have the opinions and recommendations of the doctor been threatened, refuted, discussed, rejected, and not followed as has been the case recently. An insidious competitor of the doctor has crept into the thoughts of the patient and his or her loved ones, pouring avalanches of data and the most contradictory readings into them. Who is this competitor? Why, no one else but Dr. Google—and he brings with him distortions, deviations, and interpretative doubts. The doctor was once a lofty figure, endowed with exclusive knowledge: science. The doctor could not be contradicted, only listened to. And his dictates were performed without hesitation or doubt. Today, the network satisfies an essential primary need, that of a patient and/or a family member to know, to understand better, to fully comprehend the situation in which they find themselves. The congestion of health systems and the consequent compression of the times available for meeting, combined with the hectic life of each one of us, greatly reduce the moment of dialogue between the patient and the doctor. As a result, loneliness and anxiety become additional stimuli for research and reading. Unfortunately, two other factors come into play at this point: the democracy of the web, and the specific cultural preparation of the patient.

The democratic nature of the network comes into play because it allows the right of citizenship to all content, attractive and ugly, useful and useless, reliable or anything but accurate. On the contrary, thanks to our many technical devices, it is highly likely that company-based and commercially oriented content has more visibility; that is, it is much more easily traceable than other content. The specific cultural preparation of the patient (combined with the difficulty of carrying out real in-depth investigation) is almost never enough to distinguish and recognize whether or not something is reliable. But the result of this breathless research, of these incomplete readings, of unreliable data or storytelling, turns, in most cases, into a veil of doubt cast over doctors, their diagnoses, and their recommendations. As a result, there is an explosion of outlets singing the praises of treatment protocols that have not been scientifically certified, and there are crusades against medical practices objectively protecting social health. Paradoxically, this phenomenon, playing itself out right in front of our eyes, is observed (and promoted) even by subjects who make the health sector their purpose of existence. The companies active in this field are all committed to creating content, articles, videos, and case histories. The result ends up feeding, even in good faith, the distorted behavior of patients. Today, more and more, doctors (and above all their opinions) are under increasing pressure. They are stuck between what can be found on the web and the relentless requests of patients, who go so far as to demand the prescription of this drug or that procedure because they have seen, read, and chatted about it. They know what they need, and they don't want the doctor to stand in the way of the solution they have found. So the doctor is left to his or her task as a notary of sorts, writing and prescribing, certifying. In times of illness or poor health, the doctor was once a salvific deity, but today he or she risks being reduced to carrying out a task, ratifying decisions that have been suggested by a blog. The doctor must therefore become aware that the digital revolution in the health sector also becomes an opportunity to regain his or her role of preeminence, of leadership. As long as he or she knows, with method and haste, how to adapt to the changes that are on their way.

Will Doctors Disappear?

Digital transformation can (and will) impact in different ways the medical profession and the role of the doctor. Some believe that the doctor will disappear or almost disappear, mainly because a whole series of activities currently in the hands of the doctor will be carried out by software or processes that will be integrated, often even entrusted to the patients themselves. And all this is one of the great topics of discussion in an attempt to predict the future. I believe that we will achieve a decisive change, a moment of major discontinuity with the past and a radical transformation of the doctor's role, without arriving at his or her disappearance but rather at an *enhancement* of the role.

A few considerations are to be made. Currently, the doctor interprets most of the information available retrospectively using a patient's medical history and past symptoms. Doctors use this as a basis for diagnostic interpretations and/or hypotheses of the diagnostic/therapeutic journey. As this takes place, the doctor also defines certain types of examinations necessary precisely to confirm the diagnosis made. This type of activity is destined to be completely overturned, undergoing a kind of reversal from the problem/symptom–solution/diagnosis paradigm. This process is essentially *acute*—the doctor or patient observes or feels something, there is a problem, and the search for a solution takes place in a one-on-one relationship between doctor and patient. Through this process the doctor relies on medical history, which is something that very often concerns the patient's memory and description of a particular symptom.

In digital health, we are transitioning away from this type of medicine. Digital health will look increasingly like something related to anticipatory aspects, to a predictive activity, based on a large amount of data available. We are moving toward a scenario where the doctor receives consent to access the patient's data, which is collected by devices, apps, and software, and made available asynchronously through platforms. With this data available, as well as the help of additional specific software and algorithms, the doctor will be able to orchestrate the therapeutic diagnostic intervention instead of making hypotheses and inferences as has been the case until now.

Diagnostic intervention will no longer simply repair a breakdown or manage a pathology, but increasingly it will anticipate any potential breakdown or possible pathology, and thus be able to prevent its harmful consequences. Or, in the case of a natural, genetic propensity to a specific pathology, significantly delay its onset. In addition, at the moment, this type of activity is individual, but the predictive and data analysis approach will make it, in most cases, multidisciplinary and multiple, with more doctors interacting in the management of each case. In fact, if patients can access this organized data, they can give access to more subjects. The one-on-one relationship with the doctor will transform itself into a real care team, with a number of skilled members who can intervene in patient problems in an integrated way. Let's imagine all this applied globally. The first great consequence will be incredible time savings for doctors, going so far as to also affect the distribution of medical personnel, allowing a simpler organizational possibility in order to compensate for the abundance or scarcity of doctors in relation to a community or territory. Another consequence is the change in the relationship with the patient support staff. The current nursing class will be equally impacted by the digital evolution, playing a much larger role than they currently do. All this will bring doctors back, precisely because of the greater availability of time, to being able to holistically and humanely manage their patients, to deal with their patients much more empathetically, and to be free from the bureaucratic administrative tasks to which they are currently obliged to dedicate the greater part of their attention.

Necessary Scientific Validation

The new role of the doctor leads to the theme of the validation of digital health interventions. Digital change in industries such as music or travel has simply taken place because of the technological capacity that enables new approaches. These advances have had to overcome the stumbling blocks of economic protectionism of the old status quo. In a sensitive sector such as health, all digital practices require scientific validation of the highest level, because they are so crucial by nature. A very strict validation is needed, as is the case with traditional drugs. After that, in order for knowledge to be shared, valid interventions are required to communicate with the medical class. Then, it will be necessary to understand how the doctor can relate to this new way of thinking and offering assistance to patients. This would lead over time to a health system more focused on the specific needs of patients, and hence, it is considered patient-centered health.

Patients as Health-Care Consumers

As previously mentioned, the Covid-19 pandemic and the resultant use of virtual care solutions are pushing toward a more personalized and affordable care model based on the needs of patients. In sectors such as travel, music, or fashion, the consumer experience has long since become central, considered the only true factor of differentiation. Today this also happens in the health world, where we are witnessing the consumerization of health care. This phenomenon is driven by the spread of digital health solutions and services that allow patients to be able to manage and control their own health. This also changes the very role of patients, who are increasingly searching for value in the health services they choose. This means that patients increasingly expect to have services tailored to their needs that are both accessible and empathic. This also means that those health-care services and providers must change their approach and design future care services in such a way as to provide patients with comfort, easier access, and a positive experience. In the future of medicine, those who create care services will also have to involve patients in the design of the various interfaces and services, exactly as in other sectors where the consumer helps to define the product and is indeed essential to that end. Precisely this process of patient involvement will be the key to having an improved path to health care.

CHAPTER 11

Old versus New
Embracing the Future

A Necessary Adaptation

What is certain is that the development of the technology will not stop. Today we already observe that the push of traditional companies (i.e., those already active in the pharmaceutical and medical equipment sector) is flanked by that of the most digital companies (i.e., those that produce software, apps, and devices). To these are added the new companies, vertical startups in the sector. This pressure for innovation will fuel people's natural desire for discovery in a self-fueling spiral of progress. The output of all this will be an evolution of aspirations and behaviors of people who will want to anticipate the possible state of illness in hopes of avoiding it.

This process is already in place all over the world. As we have seen in the previous chapters, wearable apps and devices already monitor and collect data on millions and millions of subjects who, voluntarily, automatically or semi-automatically, are building an image of their health that is updated in real time. But while all this is already happening around us, what seems to remain immutable is the figure of the doctor. Of course, new doctors will have to be educated and trained in the new medicine. But at the moment, neither the university nor training courses are going in the direction of digital health. This is a major problem. It is a direct problem for doctors because, without proper preparation, they are destined to lose authority in the relationship with the patient. At the same time, it poses a complication for patients, who find themselves having to do without an enlightened guide and the related support.

If we look at the two situations, it would seem that we can deduce that in fact the doctor's situation is by far the more precarious and compromised one. The weakness of the position is twofold. On the one hand, the doctor is left alone to face the colossal paradigm shift that is emerging, and which will be asserted in a short time. On the other hand, the possibility of changing one's situation necessarily involves realities and institutions, such as universities, national health services, and large private hospitals. These are very complex and bureaucratic ecosystems, upon which the doctor (even in an associated form, as a national order and/or professional category) does not have the necessary strength for making an impact.

New Training

Training is very important, indeed essential in governing or partici-
pating in digital transformation. Today, within the academic journey,
no actual cultural and technical training of this sort occurs; there is
simply no digital training. There is not a single text, not even one
exam. Even in the necessary years of postgraduate training to undertake a specialization, there is no approach, no practical experimentation. At the moment, the medical field's best hope is likely some
volunteer, perhaps motivated by a personal passion for digital issues,
and who is somehow able to keep pace with the times. But serious
problems arise from the lack of an overall vision, the absence of the
necessary systematic approach, and the fact that the solution is absolutely insufficient from a numerical point of view. Otherwise, today it
would make a lot of sense to introduce specific teachings on a whole
range of technological issues, and probably (and I say this without
too much fear) eliminate or reduce training on issues that are already
dated by the time the doctor is practicing the profession. I believe
that doctors will play a huge role in the future, but just to be clear,
their role will be very different from their role today. Take the case
of diagnostic imaging. Being good at this type of diagnostic exam
requires lengthy experience, having seen a huge number of images,
knowing how to correlate them with the diagnoses, and being able
to recognize problems and causes at a glance. But no doctor can beat
image-recognition software that has stored 10 million images and can
correlate them with proven diagnoses and cross-reference them. This
is simply because a doctor can't see and learn the same quantity of
data as a machine can. In the near future, programs of this kind will
have fewer medical specializations of that sort. Instead, doctors may
specialize, for example, in the ability to create a relationship and
help patients get untangled from a whole series of processes that by
the very nature of technology become increasingly complex.

Over time, training has become necessary not only related to
digital health, but also in the ways that, bit by bit, the profession and
medical activity have evolved over time.

There are apps that ensure that medical teams can better manage their workflow, securely collaborate on patients' treatments, and

discuss challenging cases with their peers. As well as having instant, direct access to colleagues working in their organization, doctors can also tap into a broader network of expertise.[1]

A Collective Effort Is Needed

This is probably the most delicate front, constituting, at the same time, one of the greatest consequences and one of the most radical transformations caused by the digital revolution in the health sector. There seem to be two main stumbling blocks: the assumption of responsibility within the "system that produces doctors," and the speed of technological change (and immediately afterwards, consequently, of social behavior). Today, even if taking into account the differences between the various countries, doctors are educated substantially in one way. First, a university training, then a specialization training related to the relative and specific inclination of the medical profession that the person has chosen. The first phase is, indeed, scholastic, while the second phase is more corporate. The biggest differences depend on how much a university follows, as an example, state directives or aims at relationships with companies to plan training that is considered acceptable. It's also important to consider how much specialization training may differ where it is carried out in the company or in a hospital, and, then, in a private hospital or one belonging to a national public health service. In any case, nothing in relation to a digital approach to health is being addressed today. This fact leads to a special challenge. Indeed, to overcome this gap, it will be necessary to have an effort that is shared, choral, almost as if it were a supply chain. Companies and universities (as is already the case in other sectors, such as engineering and mechatronics) will have to work side by side, collaborating and throwing all their energy into overcoming the obstacles. Given the delicacy of the medical sector, which is always under the watchful, but encouraging, gaze of the state authority, this is even more necessary. The challenge is also twofold. In fact, it is not only a question of training new doctors in a new, better oriented way, but also (and perhaps mostly) updating those who are already doctors. Two very different routes will require different approaches.

Note

1. Editorial Team. "Dutch Tinder rival app 'The Inner Circle' now available in Hong Kong, Sydney and Melbourne," *Silicon Canals*, October 4, 2018. Available at: https://siliconcanals.com/news/startups/dutch-tinder-rival-app-the-inner-circle-now-available-in-hong-kong-sydney-and-melbourne/.

CHAPTER 12

Trust versus Fear
The Path Ahead

The Horizon Opening Before Us

This digital health revolution opens up many new questions. Fundamentally, the cornerstone that sees the greatest paradigm changes is represented by the greater amount of data that will be available concerning an individual person. When this data is collected and made available, a profound change will be triggered, (as we have seen, medicine becomes predictive), which has an impact on legal and ethical issues that will have to be addressed and resolved. From a purely practical point of view, the data concerning a patient will be in the hands of the patient himself or herself. Basically, it will be the patient who will collect the data items directly and store them. After that, he or she will allow access to this data to a doctor, a hospital, multiple doctors, an athletic trainer, nutritionist, dietitian, and so on. Thus, patients will be creating their own care teams, who will make step-by-step recommendations, pointing out any misalignments with a state of good health. (The data will, obviously, be calibrated to the person's age, gender, activities, goals, and so on.) The care team will bring along suggestions and therapies to preserve the state of good health for as long as possible.

Even with a digital approach to health, the theme of trust in the relationship between the patient and every member of the care-team will be fundamental. Trust in the skills of the therapist, but also in the relational and operational mechanism being established. Because, obviously, there is also the issue of privacy. This huge amount of data must be treated with a sensitivity and delicacy that extends to all connected behaviors, which must be refined. The legal part and the ethical part are completely new. For example, some ethical problems will arise that today we can only imagine, but which instead will have their own topicality. From the management of emergencies to that of the transplant lists, such issues will affect also the availability and allocation of treatment resources. Another example can be foreshadowed when we have environmental data interpolated with genetic data, so as to have a picture of the onset and course of diseases, thus arriving at legal, ethical, and political administration issues that will have to be managed simultaneously.

In some countries, such as the United States, the process of digitizing and using data from the clinical records started earlier than in other countries, and there is currently a very heated debate on this issue. The question arises as to whether patients should have the ability to safely get hold of their data at any time from the electronic medical record system, even the kind of data that the various care providers generally jealously keep to themselves. This question leads to another: Should the computerized medical record be open to all organizations requesting consultation, or should there be some freely available data and other data that is instead specific and owned by a given platform? A solution will have to be found to all these questions, not only in the United States, but throughout the world. A balance will have to be struck between the various positions, but I also believe that, in order to be able to manage and use them in the development of solutions for the common good, there will have to be assurance that a large part of the important information must be available and open and, certainly, be fully available to the patient from whence it comes.

Today, we all have a digital fingerprint. For example, as we surf the web, we see a banner of exactly the shoes we had in mind, just the ones we were looking for, maybe at a discounted price. This does not seem strange to us anymore, although we did find it strange years ago; perhaps by now it even suits us quite well. These are the wonders of continuous profiling. And what if the same thing happens in health? What if at some point a banner appeared asking, "Are you worried about your tremor?" and clicking on it I had access to a rigorous and scientifically approved test? After that, I could be reassured by the result of the test or be advised to book a specialist visit or video consultation with a remote doctor (at an acceptable price), without the obligation of going to a doctor's office and maybe spending much more. What would I think of such a thing? Would that bother me? Would that scare me? Or would I find it convenient and think it was a good thing, given the undoubted advantages? This is, of course, a matter that needs to be subjected to regulation, but I would like to say not only that this scenario will indeed happen, but that it will also be something positive.

Double face medal

Let's draw a parallel and think about car insurance. I was born in Naples and lived there until I was 20 years old. I remember one day I received a letter from my insurance company telling me that at the end of the day, the policy would no longer be renewed at the same price as the previous year. Instead, it would be renewed at a much higher rate. I asked for an explanation since I was never involved in an accident. They told me that statistically there had been so many accidents in my area that even I could cause one in the coming year, which increased my insurance risk. Although the reasoning was not particularly brilliant, I had to renew at a price four times higher than a motorist who lived a few kilometers away. Now let's imagine a similar scenario involving health insurance. If an insurance company told you that instead of obtaining coverage for a particular price (perhaps exorbitant, since it is based on the statistics and life expectancy of people of your gender and age), it could insure you at a much fairer and cheaper price, as long as you wear a wearable device and use a given app that actually demonstrates how much physical activity you do and what type of nutrition you follow. What would you do?

Well, I'd go for the wearable. That's kind of what happens with people agreeing to install a black box in their car to get a more affordable premium for car insurance. Now let's think about the parallel situation with health insurance. As we have seen, digital health medicine will be predictive, because it can be based on ever lower costs due to the analysis of genetic predispositions.

Perhaps it would be possible to determine that a certain person is highly predisposed to pathologies of the cardiovascular system. Knowing this in advance, a health-care team will be able to advise the subject regarding nutrition, physical activity, and monitoring. In this way, the risk of the onset of the pathology will be lowered and, if it still appears, it may have a lower level of severity. However, in the same situation, a person could be charged a higher cost for health insurance after sharing their data with the insurance company, precisely because he or she is predisposed to a certain pathology. This could lead to the problem of some people not being able to find any company willing to insure them, or they may face insurance premiums so high that they are not affordable or practical.

CHAPTER 13

Exponential versus Incremental

The Unstoppable Digital Transformation of Health

A Financial Revolution Too

Due to their strategic nature, the areas of health, personal care, and medical care in general have always involved a high concentration of economic interests. Since ancient times, the use of the powers of a shaman, a sorcerer, or some other healer has never seen any limitations because, when a life was at stake, everything was done to find the means necessary to pay for healing. The relationship between wealth and the possibility of salvation has always been very closely connected. It was only with the century of the Enlightenment, and the subsequent 19th-century wave of the formation of nations (at least as far as the Western world is concerned), that the first projects of global health care of a population by a state entity had their beginning. The structure of various national health services, as they have developed to this day, took place mainly in the second half of the 19th century. But it was precisely this assertion and development of national health services that led to the excessive growth of a health-care economy that ended up giving life to large companies, giants dedicated to the production of medical devices, as well as to logistical and specialist supply chains. Currently, this is a market worth trillions of dollars as a whole, but purely economic data alone is not able to fully explain its value. Strategy and politics are two factors that should not be underestimated. Modernity has seen major advances in the evolution of the ability to cure people (e.g., vaccines, antibiotics, etc.). This emerged alongside the development of a greater capacity for food production, which was the cornerstone of population growth and the increase in life expectancy. All this has led to the fact that the world's population has reached 7.8 billion during 2020. Leading demographers believe that by 2050, we can expect a further increase of 25 percent, for a total of 9.9 billion people on the planet.[1] This figure is so gigantic that it cannot but influence politics, the economy, industry, and, of course, the health sector. Health is a concept that is totally transversal in its interest, giving it the same significance in our lives as gender, religion, nationality, age, and socioeconomic status. That is, health affects everyone, always, everywhere, and in all cases. The Covid-19 pandemic has indeed turned this into public knowledge and this further qualitative leap will bring even more geopolitical changes in the years to come.

This makes it a key area that sees the interest stratified from the individual to the family unit, from a territory to a nation, from a continent to the entire assembly of nations. Therefore, considering the refining of logistics, the speed of globalization, and the growth of wealth in nations that until the last century had been considered poor, a revolutionary concept is emerging. This is happening simply because health is so expansive. The market for a drug is global for the simple reason that any pathology is the same all over the world. Until now such an industry could produce a drug and distribute it only where agreements or logistics allowed. Now, with technology and the global market, a drug can reach every corner of the earth. As technology progresses, exports will not be limited to only products such as drugs, medical devices, or equipment; the services of a health-care company or even of the individual doctor can also be delivered to distant places. If we look at the simple economic consequences of all this, we can easily see how the growth is potentially enormous. This whets the appetite of many. Hence, there is a race among those who are already operating in the sector to delineate market perimeters and grab growth areas. There is also the tendency of new players to enter into this expanding market, whether they are financial or industrial in nature.

It is obvious that being able to guarantee a high standard of care to a population means determining the health and strength of that nation. This is the political level underlying the health-care sector, and it can only exponentially increase its economic value. Health has always been a politically and economically strategic sector, but until now, it has grown incrementally, comparable to what has taken place in other industrial sectors. The impact of digital technologies (and the cultural change that it induces in people and societies) will spur economic growth. The first effects are already being seen, but there will also be political and strategic growth that is no longer incremental but exponential. It is a bit like when you go to compare the turnover and number of employees of a giant like Walmart or Facebook. For example, you may discover that Facebook's turnover is double or triple that of Walmart. This is also what will happen with the evolution of the health sector around the world. The disruption generated by the digital revolution will lead to the birth of start-ups destined to become giants, and the current giants, if they hope to maintain their preeminence, will have to have the intelligence to comprehend the moment we are living in.

Digital Health-Care Investments around the World

Thanks to a dramatic shift to virtual health care during the Covid-19 pandemic, investment in telemedicine solutions nearly tripled between 2019 and 2020, growing from $1.1 billion to $3.1 billion, and the number of deals doubled. According to StartUp Health Insights, the funds invested in remote monitoring companies doubled over the same period, from $417 million to $941 million. We also saw a significant increase in funding in mental health with investment in the sector more than doubling from $599 million in 2019 to $1.4 billion in 2020.[2]

Also thanks to digital technologies, the way we understand health is changing. Digital health is the key concept of this transformation, in which the reference models, objectives, expectations, and more generally, the vision, are changing.

The health sector has begun a radical digital transformation in the same way, and perhaps more so than what can be seen in other industries in recent years. Digital health represents a real revolution because it allows all players in the sector to redesign the production processes and how to deliver health-care services. It is also changing the ways in which users themselves are involved.

In this context, even the patients (i.e., all of us) evolve and, thanks to technology, they become more and more active in managing their own health. Seventy-seven percent already use technology for the care of their well-being, and 55 percent are willing to share their health data through devices with interlocutors in the sector and insurance companies. This trust allows us to regain our social role, together with excellence of digital health and other players in the health world, making products more accessible and raising people's awareness on the prevention and care of their own well-being.

What has been seen in recent years has been steady and unstoppable growth. The industry's economic story begins in 2010, when, with 153 projects financed, the global value of investments was a mere $1.2 billion. Values increased in 2011, when $2 billion was invested in 283 projects. This became $2.3 billion (across 476 projects) in 2012, before rising to $2.9 billion (across 647 projects) in 2013. There was a decrease in projects financed in 2014 (608) but there was a substantial increase in the overall economic value. That year, the industry was valued at $7.1 billion, more than double the value of the previous year. Recovery began in 2016 when $6.4 billion was invested in 684 projects. This trend continued in 2017, when there were 851 projects (a record number), with an investment of $11.7 billion. The following year the number of projects dropped to 765 but recorded investments of $14.6 billion. In 2019, the number of projects was slightly lower (727) and the funds invested amounted to $13.7 billion.

We finished 2020 with a colossal $21.6 billion raised globally across every sector of health innovation. That makes 2020 the most-funded year in history for health tech. That year bested 2019 by 55 percent and 2018 by 46 percent.[3] (See Figure 13.1.)

In 2020 we saw an increase in funding for virtual care and telehealth startups, research and development virtualization, and digital therapies. In particular, in the sectors of data analytics, mHealth, clinical decision support, practice management solutions, wearable sensors, wellness, health-care booking, and social health networks saw increases in funding.

Outside the United States, the most funded hubs are China, the United Kingdom, and Israel. With 39 deals in 2020, London ranks as the most active health innovation hub. While the coronavirus slowed down Chinese investing for six months, Beijing, Guangzhou, and Hangzhou are back on the leaderboard.[4]

In 2020, the APAC digital health ecosystem closed at $6.14 billion in venture capital funding, 25 percent higher as compared to 2019. With just $1.39 billion invested, the impact of Covid-19 on the Chinese economy saw the first six months of the year in APAC at its lowest venture-capital performance since 2016, down 57 percent as compared to the first half of 2019. With the reopening of the national economy in China in the second half of the year, a strong uptick in investment activity in the third and fourth quarter resulted in the largest quarters in history as well as 17 mega-deals, a new record!

Overall, China accounted for $4.93 billion or 80 percent of the venture capital funding in APAC in 2020, up 50 percent year over year (YOY). Other subregions in APAC saw investments decreasing, with South Asia at $476 million, down 40 percent YOY; North East Asia at $392 million, down 23 percent YOY; and South East Asia at $244 million, down 5 percent YOY. Investment in Oceania increased by 50 percent YOY to $104 million.

Health Innovation Funding Year Over Year

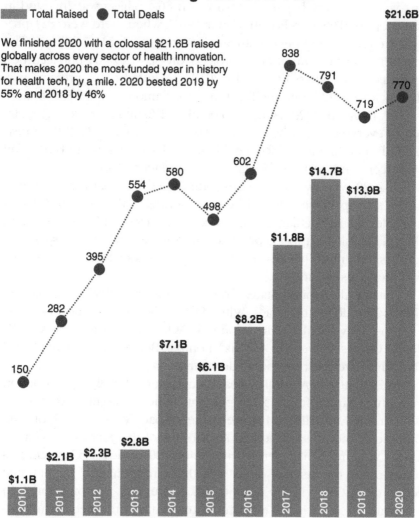

We finished 2020 with a colossal $21.6B raised globally across every sector of health innovation. That makes 2020 the most-funded year in history for health tech, by a mile. 2020 bested 2019 by 55% and 2018 by 46%

Source: StartUp Health Insights l startuphealth.com/insights. Note: Report based on publicity available data through 12/31/20 on seed (incl. accelerator), venture, corporate venture, and private equity funding only. Companies tracked in StartUp Health Insights may fall under multiple moonshots and therefore will be represented throughout the report.

FIGURE 13.1 Funding Snapshot: Year Over Year

With early and growth-stage investment decreasing as compared to 2019, venture capital across Series D and later stages accelerated, concentrating 45 percent of the total venture funding invested in 2020. The total investment value across these late-stage deals increased by a whopping 286 percent. Under the weight of the $3.5 billion initial public offering (IPO) by JD Health, the total deal value in digital health in APAC continues to increase, closing at $10.65 billion, double 2019.

With more than $3.0 billion or 49 percent of the total deal value share invested, medical diagnostics, online marketplaces, and health management solutions represented the most attractive digital health category clusters in APAC in 2020.[5]

At the individual country level, the United States and China are the nations that move the greatest investment flows, and this is for two fundamental reasons. First, America is the global driving force behind the digital innovations (if you take into consideration merely the concentration of tech companies in Silicon Valley). It is led by giants such as Amazon, Apple, and Google, while China once again shows that it has a good eye for technological trends and considers digital health as strategic for its socioeconomic development.

An example of this is Tencent, the Chinese technology giant, which since 2014 has transformed the Chinese insurance market by increasing its participation in terms of investments, acquisitions, and mergers. Tencent is expected to continue to invest in retail pharmacies, medical information technology, pet health care, insurance technology, medical equipment, gene therapy, gene sequencing, and other fields.

China is becoming a driver of innovation, and there is more than one analyst who thinks that the tech market, in terms of project development and product launch, will soon see the leadership shift in favor of the Asian giant, to the detriment of the United States.

America, or rather, the American giants, are not just sitting back idly. Recent news is that of the expansion of Jeff Bezos' empire into the pharma sector with Amazon Pharmacy, a virtual drug-store open only in the United States, which allows users to complete an entire transaction on their mobile devices through the Amazon app.

It's no secret that both Apple and Google have long focused their attention on the digital health market. For over 10 years, there has been a war to determine which of their respective smartphone platforms would be the one to lead the market. Apple received U.S. Food and Drug Administration (FDA) clearance for an updated version of its electrocardiogram (ECG) feature, which can identify atrial fibrillation with high heart rate, and launched its fitness platform Apple Fitness+ (see Chapter 1).

Google invested in AI platforms Wysa (chatbot) and Tempus (real-world evidence). They also launched: Google Health Studies, a mobile app for clinical research; Healthcare Interoperability Readiness Program, a cloud-based program for health-care organizations; and two AI tools to analyze unstructured medical text. All while announcing a six-year partnership with Highmark Health, and another partnership with U.S. Department of Health and Human Services (HHS) for a pilot program to help patients plan for future medical appointments.[6]

Microsoft did not stand still and launched Microsoft Cloud for Healthcare and a Covid-19 vaccine management platform with Accenture, Avanade, EY, and Mazik Global. It also announced a partnership with Sensyne Health to develop clinical AI and health cloud capabilities.[7]

In addition to the ongoing Covid-19 pandemic, 2020 has been dotted with devastation: violent fires, record-breaking unemployment, and growing inequality. But despite all this, a number of companies operating in the health technology sector continue to be listed on the stock markets.

Seven companies that were listed on the stock markets in 2020 include: primary-care startup One Medical, which raised $245 million in its January IPO; drug-discovery software company Schrodinger, which raised $232 million in a February IPO; benefits-navigation platform Accolade, which debuted in early July, raising $220 million; GoHealth, an online insurance broker that raised $916 million in its July IPO; Oak Street Health, which operates primary care centers for Medicare patients, and went public in August, raising $328 million; portable dialysis machine company Outset Medical, which raised $242 million in a recent IPO; and Amwell, a telehealth company that went public in early 2021, raising $742 million.

A Glance toward the Future

According to a report by Allied Market Research, the turnover of digital therapeutics in 2027 will reach $13.80 billion (in 2019 it was $2.88 billion).[8]

The main driving force for investments in this direction will be, above all, the need to combat rising health costs, but also the increase in the incidence of chronic diseases in the world population and, in any case, the consumerization of health as described earlier in this book. According to this analysis, the Asia-Pacific region will be the one that will show the highest compounded annual growth rate in the coming years. It may seem strange but treating oneself with an app or software will become increasingly simple, thanks to digital therapies. This new generation of therapies can have diverse advantages over the entire health-care system, not only from the point of view of economic sustainability, but from the point of view of primary prevention, which can become more effective and in many cases can contribute to reducing the onset of certain diseases. The real revolution of digital therapies is that they are designed to be focused on the needs of the patient and above all are scientifically validated with the same rigor that is used for the validation of drugs. They therefore enable a whole new dimension of medicine.

For pharmaceutical companies, digital therapies represent an opportunity for differentiating their offer and at the same time provide a chance for them to offer customized solutions that favor greater adherence to the existing drugs and better clinical outcomes.

In essence, the road seems to be mapped out. All that remains now is to follow it.

Notes

1. Population Reference Bureau. "2020 World Population Data Sheet," PRB.org, July 2020. Available at: https://www.prb.org/2020-world-population-data-sheet/.
2. StartUp Health. "StartUp Health Insights Report," StartUpHealth.com, 2020. Available at: https://www.startuphealth.com/2020-yearend-insights-report.
3. Ibid.

4. Ibid.
5. Galen Growth Asia Health Tech Intelligence. "2020 year-end global digital health report: Another record-breaking year," January 2021. Available at: https://julien-desalaberry.medium.com/2020-year-end-global-digital-health-report-another-record-breaking-year-e2143af4a0c9.
6. CB Insights. "State of healthcare report: Investment & sector Trends to Watch," January 20, 2021. Available at: https://www.cbinsights.com/research/report/healthcare-trends-q4-2020/.
7. Ibid.
8. Allied market Research. "Digital therapeutics market expected to reach $13.80 billion by 2027," press release, September 2020. Available at: https://www.alliedmarketresearch.com/press-release/digital-therapeutics-market.html.

A Radical Shift

Connecting the dots

To sum up the many reflections that have been made so far is not a simple operation, but it is not impossible, either. Rather than inferring conclusions, it is above all a question of connecting the dots and observing, not without wonder, the figure that appears. It is a very different figure from the one currently known to us when imagining the concept of health care. We are dealing with a total paradigm shift, a true revolution that will also be technological, but not completely. The true (and most complex) transformation will have to be mental and cultural. Even if the trigger is driven by digital, the real node will be human because the deepest change must be human. And, even if it is kicked off from the insiders in the sector, humans will be central actors in the story. All of us will contribute to extending, speeding up, and completing this revolution.

A strange concept which shouldn't go unnoticed is precisely due to the very nature of a change originating from the adoption of digital logics. One of the basic features of digital processes is that they operate on large numbers of users, and this fact implies that the arrival of change is inevitable for each of us. That is, this change will announce itself, be manifested, and will take place regardless of our individual will. Whether we like it or not, we will have to deal with it.

At the moment, we could almost carry it to an extreme by saying that no one is too ill or too old to ignore it. At the same time, by always realizing and leveraging the nature of a change driven by digital logics, each of us can be a part of it and drive it simply by adopting a new behavior, downloading an app, or using a data-detection tool. Therefore, we can choose whether or not to undergo this transformation or become, in our own small way, active participants. We can study it, informing ourselves about it, encouraging it, taking advantage of it. We can even take it to the point of demanding that it be used by putting pressure on the doctor, on the health facility, on the public administrator called to decide about its use.

Five Big Changes for a Paradigm Shift

The radical change that is about to take place in the health ecosystem can be divided and distinguished into five distinct revolutions. These revolutions are the essence of the paradigm shift that we are approaching and in which we will all participate. The five revolutions will have different speeds and will be realized in parallel, but they also interact with and influence one other. It may not be easy to distinguish them, but they sum up the cultural and innovation effort that is necessary. Seeing them in detail, we can realize how these are in fact characteristics of medicine, as we know it today, that are then compared to the qualities that it will soon have, thanks to the digital approach to health. So we can analyze them one by one, based on the comparison of what medicine *was* with what we assume it will be.

Acute versus Preventive

Today all medicine is *acute*. Even when we consider chronic conditions, we focus on emergency situations. *Chronic* describes the patient's situation, which forces him or her to live with a condition and consider it "normal." When this chronic situation is complicated by a pathological peak, the patient experiences an acute situation. Often, this is considered an emergency that causes the patient to turn to medicine for help. Today's medicine is designed around *ex-post* interventions of an event. In fact, the language of today's medicine reflects this aspect. The doctor starts from the medical history, that is from the patient's memory of what happened. The medicine of the future, in contrast, will be preventive. Since it is based on the analysis of data and predispositions, tomorrow's medicine must concern itself with improving our quality of life and delaying or preventing a whole series of diseases.

Observational versus Data Driven

Today, medicine is still based on observation of the patient and what may have occurred to him or her. Even when carrying out laboratory tests or diagnostic imaging, a part of an infinitely more complex system is observed. In the future, every person will be able to automatically or semi automatically collect a large amount of their own data concerning them, and do so in a way that this data is analyzed in real time, in order to report any significant changes.

One-by-One versus Collectively

We are already collecting results and medical histories dedicated to all pathologies and including it medical literature. But when a patient is treated, reference is only made to his or her specific situation. Imagine how much more defined the picture of the situation could be if, thanks to the consultation and filtering of homogeneous data, universally collected, it were possible to access thousands of similar situations in real time.

Retrospective versus Predictive

In the coming years, genetic analysis will be easier and cheaper. So, this will bring about the end of questions about the health of parents and grandparents in order to try to have an intuition and imagine a sort of medical history. As genomics progresses, it will be very easy to know what kind of pathologies we are more susceptible to, and then implement preventive safeguards, behaviors, and precautions. If a pathology proves inevitable due to our extreme predisposition, we will have a series of aids, stimuli, and insights to better understand and manage the problem.

Fragmented versus Integrated

As already mentioned, the five revolutions are different but interacting, and probably their interconnected nature is best understood by analyzing this specific paradigm shift. As a rule, today, in normal times, a person does not treat himself or herself. When something goes wrong with the body, when there is a breakdown or pain, the person takes action and resorts to going to the doctor. It's a bit like bringing a car to the body shop. For a dented door, a car goes to the auto-body shop; for faulty wiring, the car goes to a motor vehicle electrician; and so forth. Similarly, a patient with an earache chooses an ear, nose, and throat doctor rather than an orthopedist. Tomorrow, however, we will have a more comprehensive, integrated approach. Thanks to predictive and preventive settings, and the continuous and constant availability of data, medicine will be more aimed at providing indications and stimuli to refine and maintain a state of good integral health that concerns all physical aspects simultaneously.

The Final Goal: Humanize Care through Technology

The most important revolution, the paradigm that will change to the nth power, is, however, another, and by its nature it is the most crucial node, but also the least obvious and predictable one. The current health systems, although very different from each other, have a common feature: they are not able to guarantee universal performance or, for the most part, are not able to do so in a practical and efficient way. Throughout the Western world, we discuss organization and health economics, while there is one universally valid condition: those who have the means to do so can cure and care for themselves, while those who have fewer means need to save money for their health care. However, any health system now finds itself having to establish, with great difficulty, a balance between the growth in the number of patients and their constant ageing, and the natural and just desire of people to age in the best possible way. The proliferation of pathological conditions and the ever-increasing public needs, always aimed at seeking the latest solutions, constitute an unsolvable challenge, primarily from a financial point of view, but also from the viewpoint of the provision of services. This is unsolvable without a real change of scenario. Changing the current dysfunctions of health-care services is possible thanks to technologies. And in the previous chapters we have seen how this is happening and will happen in various specific sectors, and above all, how this will happen in our mentality, in the way we think about and approach this challenge. But thanks to the technologies available, there will also be another change, a direct consequence of the restructuring of services, but probably even more epochal: thanks to these technologies, health services will also become more humane, recovering a level of empathy never reached in the last century. A couple of examples can help us understand.

In a world where one can book low-cost flights or choose a hotel room thanks to a (banal but evolved) booking platform, health-care waiting lists simply no longer have the right to citizenship. It would be enough for every CT or MRI machine (but the example applies to other resources, from an operating room to a dialysis machine) to be connected to the network. (Do we not hear every day about IoT, the Internet of Things?) This would make it possible to check when there are moments when nothing is available and others when it is possible to allow people to book their appointments. This is already happening within the health services, with cumbersome and, above all, closed mechanisms, ones that are not in dialogue with each other. If this opening were to take place (and it will take place), soon enough someone will develop an independent platform for booking health-care services and making appointments (and who knows whether or not some startups have already done so just while you are reading these lines?). What would that mean for us? Waiting for availability is, frankly, demoralizing. Each of us could find the nearest available CT, both in the sense of kilometers and calendar days. Perhaps a patient can travel a little farther to get a test or examination without having to wait. This would also facilitate the comparison between like technologies with regard to the quality of the service and its costs, thus helping to create a reputation-based competition between various centers, which would be entirely to the benefit of those who use the services. A person's health, just like his or her social network, is affected by a number of aspects, such as income, place of birth and residence, literacy, and so forth. When a person has a health problem, the basic reaction is the activation of the social network, asking family members, friends, and other trusted people for recommendations for doctors. These practices allow one, relatively quickly, to get to the appropriate doctor for the current problem, perhaps even skip some queues because someone in our social network presents this person to us and introduces us. In this case, the expectation of healing is quite high. But it is very different from the expectation of a person who, after the appearance of a problem, waits a few weeks, because he or she is not sure about the symptoms, and then decides to see the general practitioner, who perhaps prescribes examinations, which then get the person to see a specialist. So, six or twelve months later, he or she is still groping in the dark, or is still, at any rate, far from the solution of the problem. That period of time can be harmful in certain pathologies and cases. Why is technology so important in this radical health transformation? Because, as the WHO has long published, the determinants of human health are only partly linked to biological aspects—after simplification—for example, to genetic aspects. Everything else that contributes is independent of this. Whatever health problems a person may have, the prognosis is influenced by a number of factors, including income and knowledge of the right place to turn to at the right time. All of us have had experiences like this and would be able to imagine it without any difficulty. For the most part, the prognosis is influenced by these aspects: the availability of the drug, accessibility, the possibility of buying it, and so forth. Very soon, however, the technologies will take care of tracking our data passively, and at the same time, they will be able to give us guidance about healthy lifestyles. In the presence of certain symptoms, they will be able to immediately push us to have the corresponding health tests, perhaps independently. From those tests, we will identify the problem and, at the same time, be put in contact with the right doctor very quickly because the availability of that doctor is optimized by a capacity management system. (A common example of this is the software used to allocate seats in an airplane.) That doctor will prescribe a therapy that can be carried out at home, thanks to the appropriate devices, which will also allow remote monitoring. So when (not if, but when, and when is very close) these technologies will allow this scenario to take place, it is evident that a health-care system will be able to provide the best care to a very large number of people (if not all) at a sustainable cost to the system.

All this will free up energies that will allow people to discuss the state of their health, to be able to communicate, to be able to receive empathy. It will allow, even in serious situations, collaboration with caregivers and health-care providers on an extremely human level, precisely because the complexity, bureaucracy, slowness, fears, anxieties, uncertainties, suboptimal procedures, lack of information, and even rudeness that afflict the current health-care system will have vanished. The intrinsic efficiency of the system will wipe out these defects, leaving room for a return to more humane health care. To sum up, everything that can become digital will surely become so. For years, since the moment I started, I've been told, *It's never going to happen, this can't be done, this thing can't be digitized, this has always worked this way.* Yet, it's going to happen as in all other industries. All the processes that can be digitized are going to be digitized. It is inexorably only a matter of timing, complexity, and due caution, but it will certainly happen. That's why I think there's going to be a radical digital health transformation, and that digital will be much more than what we see today. It's going to be a truly transformative force in health care in the deepest sense.

Everything I am doing and trying to do, together with the team that supports me in Healthware, regardless of whether we are accompanying newborn startups, or carrying out consultancy for huge multinational companies engaged in innovation and transformation, is written here.

All this only makes sense if you are able to break the equation of failure of health care, of health as we know it today. The need for health care is much greater than what we can deliver, and it is unsustainable economically, regardless of the structure of the system. With the current paradigms, it is not possible to give the best standard of care to all those who need it, regardless of any economic aspects, because it is simply not sustainable.

In our vision, digital health should make all of this possible. How? By creating huge efficiencies on different processes. Consequently, those efficiencies and the resulting solutions will make it possible to solve this equation and make the best standards of care accessible to everyone, whenever and wherever it is needed. This will recover the humanization of health care, removing from the equation all bureaucracy aspects of the process, economic waste, and dysfunction that the system that even in its best versions is plagued by nowadays. And this is what we hope for with regard to the real deployment of digital health.

More humane and more democratic because:

- By removing complications, waste of time, and bureaucracy (which from the patient's point of view are painful), and making health-care systems more efficient, technology allows the doctor to focus as much as possible on the direct relationship with the patient or on empathy, which is as important as science in the care of people.
- By making systems more efficient, care will cost less. This will lead to more democracy and equality (*mutatis mutandis*, the things that need to be changed have been changed). To borrow an example from the airline industry, one can think of how the introduction of low-cost fares has led to the significant expansion of the air transport user base. In the case of digital health, there will be no distinction between high and low prices, because the costs will fall for everyone.
- Creating a doctor-patient relationship based on science and empathy will allow the patient to better understand the type of care he or she is receiving, becoming an active part of this process through self-help and helping those around him or her, whether they are family members or other patients.

Here, too, the Covid-19 pandemic has shown us these phenomena in all their magnitude. How would we have been able to resist without online health information and remote support systems for both communication and case management? Of course, we could have been much more prepared and reduced the suffering and economic impact a great deal, but we have certainly learned the enormous potential of innovative health, and we should be more prepared in the future, and prepared to apply what we have learned to all other human diseases.

What's Next?

In recent times we have been able to see the rapid adoption of digital technologies in all areas of health care, thus generating several opportunities for a systemic change in national health-care systems.

This means that there will also be major changes for all the different players operating in the world of health, but it is possible to identify trends that will have greater importance in the coming months and years. A selection of the changes[1] that will have the most impact follows.

Telehealth keeps maturing and integrates into care pathways.

The adoption of telehealth, which was already accelerating pre-pandemic, has been exponentially driven by Covid-19. It's swept aside several historic barriers, such as the desire of health-care professionals and patients to physically meet, medical guidelines that focus on in-person diagnosis, and reimbursement models that discourage remote consultation.

Covid-19 made 2020 a psychological and systemic tipping point for telehealth. Its adoption will accelerate in 2021 as it becomes the norm. And in the process it will drive new self-service approaches to medicine and participation-based reimbursement models.

Mental health worsens but digital tools continue to fill the gap.

The emotional and psychological well-being of the world's population has been put under tremendous strain because of the Covid-19 pandemic, exacerbating an existing global mental health epidemic.

There is an opportunity to address this at scale with digital tools and techniques and expand support into just about any therapeutic area through the holistic integration of mental and behavioral health solutions that improve patient care.

Mental health support is key to improving outcomes in chronic diseases and can also provide an invaluable empathetic and psychological component of support for people dealing with other complex medical situations.

When coupled with conversational interfaces and AI, digital mental health solutions are perceived as highly personal by users and open the door for a profound transformation in people's relationships with digital health tools and how they integrate them into their daily lives.

Clinical trials get more and more digitalized.

As study enrollment continues to lag drastically behind targets, patient recruitment is set to rely even more on digital marketing to improve its speed and accuracy. These techniques will also need to be applied to screening, interviews, and the actual studies themselves, particularly as more trials move toward a virtual, decentralized, or hybrid model.

Digital screening of subjects makes their geographical location less relevant, which may make studies more attractive as there is less requirement to travel. And with the support of remote sampling, and growing tools for gathering real-world evidence about improved quality of life, the clinical trials of the future can be done faster, with lower costs and on a more decentralized basis.

Aging in place becomes more commonplace.

Aging in place will become more common as the Baby Boomer generation feels more comfortable leveraging tools like remote monitoring, telehealth, and disease management platforms. Living independently will be critical to this age group and digital health tools will be critical in supporting them in this endeavor. The adoption and growth of digital tools is expected to explode as a result. This is certainly evident in the amount of investment in the category.

Inevitable invisibility of digital health.

Technology will begin to dematerialize, as has already been seen in other industries, and digital health will increasingly be woven into everyday objects. We're starting to see this happen through the emergence of smart homes and smart cars (i.e., steering wheels that also measure the driver's heart rate). As more data is collected passively, there will be more opportunities for integration.

No more "business as usual" for pharma's customer engagement.

Life sciences companies need to rethink their customer engagement paradigms in light of changing customer preferences.

Pharma should update the role of the rep from simply delivering a sales message to more of a concierge service model, providing access to—and facilitating the delivery of—meaningful content that physicians want and need. As such, reps will need to be reskilled.

Self-service models for health-care plans are also needed in order to provide access to content when and how they want it; as already seen in other industries, the expectation will be for 24/7 access.

While digital-only product promotion was laughed at just a year ago, we've already seen the first digital-only blockbuster launch, and we expect this will become a growing trend. Pharma companies will need to continually rethink what works and not be afraid to experiment with solutions they've never tried before.

The need for digital health proficiency will grow.

While 2014 is often quoted as the first year where the majority of working health-care professionals were digital natives, 2020 was the year when the remaining digital immigrants were forced to travel into the online world. Post-pandemic, online engagement will continue to be commonplace and 2021 will see much broader rollouts of digital training for medics (young and old), and all medical societies will have to embrace online learning and digital publishing models. In addition, the subject matter for ongoing disease research will focus even further on Covid-19 comorbidities and the longer-term impact of the virus.

Telehealth strategy will be integrated into commercial models.

Amazon is making a serious global move into health-care delivery with the acquisition of PillPack and its recent launch of Amazon Pharmacy. With Amazon Care, it is starting to experiment with virtual health-care services, offering them first to its own employees and with plans to expand them to health plans and other employers.

These moves are bringing Amazon closer and closer to a true end-to-end model, similar to the turnkey solutions offered by the likes of Hims, Ro, and others in the category with an original focus on conditions with an associated stigma. We're already starting to see some pharma build end-to-end solutions like this in birth control, and we're expecting to see these efforts branch out into other disease areas. Beyond building end-to-end solutions like this to drive scripts, we expect pharma to begin approaching telehealth more generally as a potential marketing/sales channel, helping to remove barriers to care, improving online visits, and even helping health-care plans understand the benefits.

Digital health platforms will consolidate.

Digital health platforms will likely see a wave of further consolidations, with a few leading platforms starting to stake out their respective positions across the health-care spectrum. This trend can be seen as a net positive, in that it will enable digital therapeutic solution developers to concentrate on building the individual vertical products that will live on these platforms.

However, issues around data ownership and sharing will need to be addressed and resolved (by way of regulations) to avoid a situation where solutions that are competitive to platform owners cannot find a way to be listed on them. Price controls will also need to be mandated to avoid the types of access taxes that are currently encountered. For example, Apple's App Store charges fees on sales to app developers (upward of 30 percent of sales collected), who have no way to sell their apps directly to iPhone users.

Services to manage and make sense of the health data explosion.

We expect to see what we call health data as a service (HDaS). As more solutions and devices generate increasing amounts of health data, there is a greater need to aggregate that data in a useful way for consumers. Consumers want and need tools to make sense of all that data. They also want to ensure they know who has access to that data, and control over where it can flow. So, we expect to see more tools supporting consumers in this way.

A Greater Responsibility

As a final reflection I go back to my opening keynote at the global digital health conference, Frontiers Health in November 2020. The theme was "Spirit, Purpose, Scale and Empathy." Thinking back to those ideas, while we are still dealing with the Covid-19 pandemic, I think they are more valid than ever.

The health innovation ecosystem is up to a huge task: transforming health care. This has never been truer and more necessary. We are holding strong through these unprecedented times as much as everyone else, but we hold a greater responsibility. As innovators, we carry the torch of science and technology and thanks to the ingenuity of the founders and the researchers, we've been always the driving force of any remarkable progress.

One year ago, we were reflecting on the sense of purpose that comes with our collective mission to improve people's health, and we were also discussing the mission of making health care more sustainable and accessible. While this stays intact, this pandemic has clarified, once again, that there is no economy, there is no society, without health. It also posed a direct threat to the already insufficient level of universal access to care that we had previously. Our purpose should therefore escalate and be complemented by a sense of urgency, able to mobilize all stakeholders to accelerate these transformational innovations; digital health innovation is by far our best option to walk through the uncharted territories ahead of us.

The pioneering years are over, the pilot years are over, too. We need to scale what works, armed with the rigor of scientific evidence but also with the aim to create the highest positive impact possible. Accrue data, learn, iterate, perfect, and do it again. Then, do it faster. The only way out of this pandemic is to go through it; we need to accelerate all possible best practices and adopt them at scale. But we need to aim even bigger; the impact of the current situation on our life is unprecedented, and it will also have significant impact on the future. Too many people lack access to care for all the other diseases and conditions which have not gone away. I used to say, "Sooner or later we will all be patients; it is inevitable and important to remember."

We are touching this first-hand, as never before. We feel the fear and uncertainty, we experience the lack of clarity, and we feel the lack of access to doctors. This is not only about the Covid-19 virus, but also about all other issues whose treatments are disrupted by the current situation. Right now, we have no idea how they will resume. We are all in this together as patients and we also know how much pressure our doctors and nurses are facing. Empathy is something we need as much as medicine. It is an integral part of the care we need and there will be no success for digital health without it. Our responsibility is greater than before.

As our industry attracts as much attention as funding, we carry the responsibility of enabling digital health much faster and ensuring a much greater access. In fact, it is no longer about health itself but is about jobs, economy, society, instruction, and our future as human beings. As innovators we should all unite, as we do with this conference. Let's join forces, mobilize the policy makers, leverage the capital, and support each other to accelerate the change we need.

I am truly honored to be part of this movement and feel blessed to be able to share this journey with all of you.

Note

1. First published as an article for Pharmaphorum https://pharma-phorum.com/digital/digital-health-trends-predictions-2021/.

Appendix

Speeches by Roberto Ascione

With over 20 years of international activity, Roberto Ascione is considered one of the leading experts in the health sector, and in particular, of the digital transformation of this industry. For this reason, he is often called to intervene at events, symposia, and conferences around the world, and is asked to carry out interventions for staff and company management. The list below provides some recordings where you can hear him as a speaker:

A Greater Responsibility

The opening keynote speech held during the Frontiers Health 2020 global conference offers reflections on the task of the health ecosystem for addressing the historic moment of the Covid-19 pandemic. Available at:
https://www.youtube.com/watch?v=uJgPtY1AFJw&feature=emb_title.

Frontiers Health Live "Fight the Pandemic"—Health in the New Normal

Keynote speech at Frontiers Health Live "Fight the Pandemic" organized in 2020. Available at:
https://www.youtube.com/watch?v=_AE1lLtUS9U&t=26s.

Born on the Wrong Side of the World—TEDxSalerno

Available at:
https://www.youtube.com/watch?v=Opstu2MBbVg&t=5s.

StartUp HealthTV 2020: Roberto Ascione, Healthware Group

Roberto Ascione talks with Unity Stoakes, StartUp Health's co-founder and managing partner, about the transformations in digital health over the past decade. Available at:
https://www.youtube.com/watch?v=g2IDEil69CA.

Webit.Festival Europe 2019

In this talk he speaks about the trends and scenario of digital therapies. Available at:
https://bit.ly/webit-dtx.

Digital Health Future

The vision of the future of digital health by Roberto Ascione, together with the 20 years of experience of Healthware. Available at:
https://www.youtube.com/watch?v=l4RGYFibQqc&t=14s.

About the Author

Roberto Ascione is a pioneer in digital health and a recognized thought leader, people-inspiring founder, serial entrepreneur, and global manager. Trained as a medical doctor and in marketing communications, his passion for medicine, computer science, and human-technology interactions have led to his lifelong commitment and dedication to the advancement and spreading of digital healthcare; he holds a strong belief that digital innovations and technology will be the most impactful drivers of change in health care.

Roberto is currently CEO at Healthware Group, a global leader in health care and digital innovation, combining innovative R&D capabilities focusing on digital medicines and digital therapeutics, with commercial and medical operations for its own products and services as well as for established and emerging life-sciences and DTx companies and other health-care stakeholders.

Roberto is also very active in the digital health ecosystem in various advisor capacities both in Europe and the United States to companies, startups, and investors; among others he has been recognized as Decade's Best Industry Leader by the Health 2.0 Conference—10 Year Global Retrospective Award in 2016, nominated Transformational Leader at The PM360 ELITE Awards, and named among the 100 Most Inspiring People by PharmaVOICE, both in 2017.

He is a founding member of the Digital Therapeutics Alliance, has been president of the HealthTech Summit, and is chairman at Frontiers Health, which emerged as one of the leading digital health conferences globally.

He is a regular keynoter at global events such as Webit, MWC, Wired Health, 4YFN, HIMMS | Health 2.0, Global Entrepreneurship Congress (GEC), TEDx, Codemotion, Upgraded Life Festival, Dublin

Tech Summit, as well as large internal events for corporations like AXA, Bayer, BNP Paribas Cardif, EY, Merck, MSD, Roche, Sanofi.

In the past 25 years Roberto has been focusing on marketing and communications, business transformation, and innovation in health and wellness: between 1997 and 2006 he founded multiple companies at the intersection of health care and technology with main exit to Publicis Groupe in 2007. He held multiple roles at Publicis Healthcare up to 2013 and was Global President at Razorfish Healthware, leading a team of 200+ people in nine countries.

When not in New York City, London, or Milan, Roberto is most likely in Salerno along the Amalfi Coast, Italy.

About Healthware

Healthware Group is a global leader in health care and digital innovation, combining innovative R&D capabilities focusing on digital medicines and digital therapeutics, with commercial and medical operations for its own products and services as well as for established and emerging life-sciences and DTx companies and other health care stakeholders.

Founded in Italy in 1997 by CEO and digital health pioneer Robrto Ascione, Healthware Group encompasses several verticals and assets, including the digital therapeutics R&D partner and product portfolio division, Healthware Therapeutics, and the digital health technology platform H.Core. Flagship commercial and medical communications team Healthware International, media management and audience engagement Healthware Engage, innovation division Healthware Labs, and virtual events specialist SWM ensure comprehensive go-to-market, scientific, and pipeline building capabilities.

Also, thanks to the corporate venture, Healthware Ventures, the Healthware Group invests—also through partnerships and collaborations—in early-stage startups with a focus on digital health platforms, telehealth, and digital therapies.

The strong vocation for innovation is also expressed through the role in Frontiers Health, the global conference on digital health, and the realization of the Healthware Life Hub, an international innovation hub dedicated to the acceleration of digital health startups, inside the Palazzo Innovazione in Salerno, Italy, where the history of an ancient convent dating from the year 1000 meets the future in a hub of talent, innovative ideas, and projects.

The strategic and pioneering choices, together with innovative management methodologies and targeted investments in research and development, have been rewarded over the years by national and international successes, recognition, and awards, including: PM360 Innovators, MM&M Top 50 Agency, Webby Awards, IKA—Interactive Key Award, Web Award, W3 Awards, Web Health Awards.

Healthware has a team of 200+ professionals with main offices in Salerno, London, New York, Milan, Helsinki, and, together with its joint venture partner Intouch Group, has a combined reach of over 1,500 people in over 15 offices in Europe, the US, and Asia.

For more information, please visit healthwaregroup.com.

Acknowledgments

A person, a professional, can study, work, update, and engage himself or herself. And the fruit of all this will be condensed into personal and professional success, but this is undoubtedly true initially. To go beyond that, to exceed the share of the result directly connected to the work, we need other ingredients, conditions that amplify the results leading to an exponential growth of the same.

The first of these ingredients is precisely . . . health. Without this, it's impossible to go anywhere. Then you need a bit of luck, as necessary as the air.

And maybe you need to compete in challenging areas like this but in an international context, which bases a lot of its judgement on the trinomial of preparation, commitment, and results rather than on various shortcuts.

All this is to say that this book really represents the synthesis of my work and my thought of the last 5 to 10 years, but this synthesis would not have been possible without a determining factor: the connection with others.

Over the years, in fact, I have been able to forge relationships with other people moved, like me, by the desire to discover, experiment, meet, measure, make mistakes, and then get up and try again. And with this approach I can say that, over time, the best result I have achieved is the great collection of meetings and collaborations (and I am aware that I am very lucky to be able to say friendships) that I have built. For this reason, working on this book, I was happy with the answers I had from the people I contacted, from the willingness to collaborate that I found.

Therefore, I can only warmly thank all the friends, from all over the world, who sent me their contributions and comments inserted in these pages. But also all those who, not included in the book, advised me, encouraged me, and spurred me on.

A special thanks then goes to Andrea Sparacino of the publishing house that published the first edition in Italian, who believed in this project, and Federico Luperi, who supported the synthesis and realization of that first edition. To which were added Sara Scarpinati, Giovanna D'Urso, and Luigi Pavia, whose contribution to the first international edition was irreplaceable.

But the greatest thanks go to my team, the people of Healthware, who collaborate and believe in me every day in a huge challenge. Without them, without a high-profile and cohesive team, no results at all can be achieved.

And in my team, let me also include my family, always an inexhaustible source of encouragement and trust, thanks to the continuous and discreet presence and that ability to unite affection, firm principles, and truths that are part of their nature.

I firmly believe that digital technologies will help us transform health in a radically positive way, but health is the most personal thing that there is and, therefore, this transformation is born and returns to people by putting them at the center. At the center of a health that is, finally, more human.

My team and I have always been working toward this goal, and every day we think about how to go a little further in this direction. So, I also thank each one of you who has read these ideas so far. With this, we like to think that our journey is now also yours in some small way.

Ad Maiora!

Index

A

Abilify MyCite, 8–9
Able, Rich, 34
Accenture, 158
Accolade, 158
Acute medicine, 162–168
ADHD, 76, 77
Aetna, 7
Aging in place, 170
Aging process, 93, 164
AI, *see* Artificial intelligence
Airbnb, 59
AKH-Vienna General Hospital, 130
Akili Interactive, 76–77
Alexa, 32–34
Algorithms, 89, 124
Almirall,103, 102
AlmirallShare, 103
Altibbi, 57–58
Alzheimer's disease, 126
Amazon, 33, 34, 157, 171–172
Amazon Care, 171
Amazon Pharmacy, 157, 171
American Hospital Association, 47
Amicomed, 75, 77–78
Amwell, 158
Andreessen Horowitz, 72
Anthem, 7
Antisense oligonucleotides, 92
Anxiety relief, 10, 79

APAC digital health ecosystem,
    155, 157
Apps, 54. *See also* Digital health
    enabling platforms
Apple, 157, 158
Apple App store, 172
Apple Health, 9, 58–59
Apple Watch, 4, 6–7, 9
Appointments:
    made through Doctolib, 60, 61
    waiting for, 56, 165
Aquinas, Thomas, 16
AR (augmented reality), 31–32, 36
Artificial intelligence (AI), 2, 17–18,
    89. *See also* Data science
    and artificial intelligence
    computer-human interfaces
        using, *see* Computer-human
        interfaces
    in future of medicine, 91–92
    in processing and using
        data, 75
    in Rose's vision of the
        future, 30
Ascione, Roberto, 72, 175–176
Asthma, 73–74
Augmented reality (AR), 31–32, 36
Automated conversation
    experiences, 20–21
Avanade, 158
AZ Damiaan hospital, 38

B

Babylon Health, 34–35
Bayer G4A, 21, 102, 104
Behavioral medicine, 45
Behavior modification, 76
Bentham, Jeremy, 30
Berlucchi, Matteo, 35
Bezos, Jeff, 33, 157
Big data:
    analysis and study of, 18–19
    in clinical genomics, 94
    critical issues with, 16–17
    and genomics, 90
    for Healthily databases, 36
    in mass screening and
        prevention, 16–18
Big Health, 127
Binaural tones/binaural
    beats, 126–127
Blood oxygen measurement, 7
Blood pressure, 75, 77–78
Blood sugar monitoring, 46
Boehringer Ingelheim, 78
Borukhovich, Eugene, 80–81
Borukhovich, Marina, 128
Brin, Sergey, 90
British Heart Foundation, 126
Brooks, Byron, 46
Brotman Baty Institute for Precision
    Medicine, 7

C

Cancer, 23, 80, 92–93, 117, 128
Capacity management system,
    165, 166
Capobianchi, Dr., 88
Car insurance, 149–150
Caskey, C. Thomas, 94
Cellarity, 94–95
Chain termination method, 86

Chesbrough, Henry, 100
Chiesi Group, 109
Chronic back pain, 79
Chronic conditions, 162
Chronic diseases, 61–62, 73
Chronic obstructive pulmonary
    disorder (COPD), 73–74, 79
Church, George, 96
The Clickometrics, 78
Click Therapeutics, 78
Clinical trials, 170
Closed innovation, 100
Coder, Megan, 82–93
Cohealo, 59–60
Collective data, 163
Collective effort, in embracing the
    future, 144
Colonoscopy, 17–18
Commercial telehealth models,
    171–172
Computation, 30
Computers, 1
Computer-human interfaces,
    29–39
    Alexa and Echo, 33–34
    Babylon Health, 34–35
    Healthily, 35–36
    HoloLens, 36
    MindMaze, 37
    PatchAi, 39
    Pepper Robot, 37–38
    Psious, 38
    Roberto's view on, 32–33
Consumerization of health
    care, 140, 159
Continuous electrocardiogram, 6
Conversa Health, 19–20
Cook, Tim, 58
COPD (chronic obstructive pulmo-
    nary disorder), 73–74, 79
Co-PRO, 39
Costs of production, 4, 5

Covid-19 (coronavirus) pandemic:
  and acceleration of digital health
    solutions/tools, 131–132
  and adoption of remote
    monitoring, 44
  detecting infections, 12
  digital innovation during, 2, 66
  and Frontiers Conferences, 105
  and investment in telemedicine,
    154
  lessons from, 133, 168
  and mental health, 169
  and move toward new care
    model, 140
  new communication tools imple-
    mented during, 55–56
  new normality generated by, 57
  Nueno on, 49
  Paginemediche services during, 63
  research on, 171
  sea change provoked by, 13
  telehealth during, 43, 44, 169
  threat to healthcare
    during, 173–174
  vaccine management platform
    in, 158
  and widespread effects of
    health, 152
Crick, Francis, 86
Cupertino, 7, 58
Customer engagement by
    pharma, 170–171
Customer experience, 66
CVS Health, 127

D

Dachis, Jeff, 24–25
Dachis Group, 24
Darcy, Alison, 26
Data, 74–75. *See also* Big data
  on cancer, 93
  collective vs. one-by-one, 163
  health data as a service, 172
  on human genome, 2
  in next-generation sequencing,
    89–90
  patients' access to, 148–149
  personal, *see* Personal data
  privacy of, 17, 148
  from VitalConnect, 48
Data-driven healthcare, 163
Data-driven medicine (DDM), 94
Data ownership and sharing, 172
Data science and artificial
    intelligence, 2, 15–27
  big data in mass screening and
    prevention, 16–18
  Conversa Health, 19–20
  Dachis on, 24–25
  Levy on, 25–26
  One Drop, 20–21, 24–25
  Roberto's view on, 18–19
  Sensely.com, 21–22
  SkinVision, 23
  Woebot Health, 25–26
DDM (data-driven medicine), 94
Debiopharm, 113–114
Deep Genomics, 91–92
Deepmind Health, 17
De Heus, Erik, 23
Depression, 31, 73, 79
Design thinking, 114–115
Devices, sensors, and signals, 3–14
  Apple Watch, 6–7
  Empatica, 8, 11–12
  HealthGo, 13–14
  Lai on, 11–12
  Proteus Digital Health, 8–9
  Qardio, 9
  Ramakrishnan on, 13–14
  Roberto's view on, 5–6
  Thync, 10
  toward invisibility of digital
    health, 4–5

Devoted Health, 7
Diabetes, 21, 24–25, 45, 46, 73,
  76, 80, 123
Diagnostic intervention, 139
Diamandis, Peter, 93
Dietary advice, 123–124, 127, 128
Digital biomarkers, 5–6
Digital drugs, 8–9
Digital fingerprints, 149
Digital Garden, 102, 103
Digital health, 154. *See also*
  specific topics
Digital Health Academy, 108
Digital health enabling platforms,
  53–69
  Altibbi, 57–58
  Apple Health, 58–59
  Cohealo, 59–60
  for connecting doctors and
    patients, remote monitoring
    systems, and management
    of therapies, 54–56
  consolidations of, 172
  DocDoc, 60
  Doctolib, 60–61
  Grandell on, 67–68
  Hasan on, 65–66
  hi.health, 61
  Livongo, 61–62
  Paginemediche, 62–63
  Roberto's vision for, 56–57
  Slujis on, 63–65
Digital health proficiency, 171
Digital health start-ups, 2
Digital pharmacies, 132
Digital technologies:
  computer-human interfaces,
    29–39
  data science and artificial
    intelligence, 15–27
  devices, sensors, and
    signals, 3–14

digital health enabling
  platforms, 53–69
digital therapeutics, 71–84
lifestyle as medicine, 121–130
open innovation and
  partnerships, 99–120
personal genomics, 85–97
rapid adoption of, 168–169
reflections on, 1–2
telemedicine and remote
  monitoring, 41–51
Digital therapeutics, 71–84
  Akili, 76–77
  Amicomed, 77–78
  Borukhovich on, 80–81
  Click Therapeutics, 78
  Coder on, 82–93
  Ginger.io, 79
  Kaia Health, 79
  origin of term, 80
  Roberto's vision for, 74–76
  turnover of, 159
  Voluntis, 80
Digital Therapeutics Alliance (DTA),
  72, 80, 82
Digital therapies (DTx), 72–74,
  82–83, 159. *See also* Digital
  therapeutics
Digital transformation of healthcare,
  75, 141–145, 167
  embracing, 141–145
  exponential vs. incremen-
    tal, 151–160
  impact of, 138–139
  inevitability of, 161–162
  trust in vs. fear of, 147–150
  worldwide investments
    in, 154–159
Direct-to-consumer genetic tests
  (DTC-GT), 95–97
DNA sequencing, 86–90
DocDoc, 60

Doctolib, 60–61
Doctors:
  competitors of, 136–138
  empowered, 135–140
  future role of, 143
  impact of digital transformation
    on, 138–139
  platforms available for, 44
  training of, 143–144
  weak position of, 142
Domino's Pizza, 118
Domotics, 33
Dover, Heinrich Wilhelm, 127
Dowe, Tanja, 112–113
Dr. Google, 136
Drugs:
  digital, 8–9
  digital pharmacies, 132
  digital prescriptions for, 35
  digital therapies replacing, 72–73
  global market for, 153
DTA, *see* Digital Therapeutics
  Alliance
DTC-GT (direct-to-consumer
  genetic tests), 95–97
DTx, *see* Digital therapies
Duffy, Sean, 45

E

ECG, *see* Electrocardiogram
Echo, 32–34
Economics of healthcare
  sector, 152–153
EDA (electrodermal activity), 8
eDevice, 13–14
Efficient care, 167, 168
Electrocardiogram (ECG):
  as Apple Watch function, 7
  continuous, 6
Electrodermal activity (EDA), 8
Empathetic robot, 37–38

Empatica, Inc., 8, 11–12
Empowerment:
  of doctors and health consumers,
    135–140
  through lifestyle as medicine,
    122. *See also* Lifestyle
    as medicine
  in traditional therapies, 122
Enchanted Objects (Rose), 30
EndeavorRx, 76–77
Endoscopic system, AI-assisted,
  17–18
Equipment rental, among
  hospitals, 59–60
The Era of Open Innovation
  (Chesbrough), 100
Espie Colin, 127, 128
Estrella, Tony, 118–119
Ethics, 30, 148
Etsimo Healthcare Ltd, 68
Eversana, 127
Experiments on Plant Hybrids
  (Mendel), 86
Exponential vs. incremental
  transformation, 151–160
  digital healthcare investments
    around the world,
    154–158
  in the future, 159
EY, 158

F

Facial expression replication, 37
Fear, 147–150
Flagship Pioneering, 94–95
Flatiron Health, 92–93
Flores, Oscar, 95–97
Foundation Medicine, 96
Frey, Brendan, 92
Frontiers Conferences, 104–105, 173
Frontiers Health, 104–105

Future:
  of healthcare, *see* Digital transfor-
    mation of healthcare
  of medicine, 91–92, 140
FutureProofing Healthcare, 119

G

Gaming experience, therapy
    delivered through, 76–77
Genetics, 88–90
  AI in understanding of data of, 17
  human genome, 86–88
  Mendel's work on, 86
Genetic analysis, 163
Genomics, 88–90, 163. *See also*
    DNA sequencing;
    Personal genomics
G4A program, 21, 102, 104
Gilbert, Walter, 86
Ginger.io, 79
GISAID database, 88
GlaxoSmithKline, 74
Gliimpse, 58
GoHealth, 158
Goldwasser, Isy, 10
Google, 90, 92, 136, 157, 158
Google Health, 17
Google Health Studies, 158
Google Home, 32–33
Gorton, Michael, 46
Grandell, Thomas, 67–68
Grants4Apps, 104. *See also* Bayer
    G4A; G4A program
Grossmann Zamora, Rafael J., 36
Guardant Health, 96
GuideWell, 109
GV, 93

H

Hames, Peter, 127–138
Hasan, Ali, 65–66

HDaS (health data as a service),
  172
Headspace, 125–126
Health, determinants of, 165, 166
HealthBuilders, 76, 93, 102, 109
Healthcare consumers, patients as,
  135–138, 140
Healthcare industry:
  current defects of, 167
  humanizing, 164–168
  paradigm shift in, 161
  revolutions in, 162–168
  value of, 154–155
Healthcare Interoperability
    Readiness Program, 158
Healthcare teams, 148
Health coaches, 122, 128
Health data as a service
  (HDaS), 172
HealthGo, 13–14
Healthily, 35–36
Health Innovation Ecosystem Fight-
    ing Covid-19, 105
Health insurance, 150
HealthKit, 59, 75
HealthTunes, 126–127, 129–130
Healthware Labs, 105–106,
  114–115, 167
Healthware Life Hub Accelerator, 106
HealthXL, 106
Heart problems, 9, 45
HGP (Human Genome Project), 86
High-level parallelism, 87
Highmark Health, 158
hi.health, 61
Hims, 172
Hinduja, 37
Holley, Robert W., 86
HoloLens, 36
Human factors in innovation:
  embracing digital transformation
    of healthcare, 141–145
  empowered doctors and health
    consumers, 135–140

exponential vs. incremental transformation, 151–160
reflections on, 131–133
trust in vs. fear, 147–150
Human genome, 1–2, 86–88. *See also* Personal genomics
Human Genome Project (HGP), 86
Humanizing care through technology, 164–168
Human Longevity, 93–94
Human-machine interaction, *see* Computer-human interfaces
Hypertension, 77–78

I

Immune response, 10
Incremental transformation, *see* Exponential vs. incremental transformation
Influenza detection, 12
Ingestible devices, 5
Ingestible drugs, 8–9
Innovation(s):
adoption of, during Covid-19 pandemic, 131–132
China as a driver of, 157
closed, 100
digital, *see* Digital technologies
hubs for, 155
human factors in, *see* Human factors in innovation
open, *see* Open innovation and partnerships
Insomnia, 73, 128
Insulia, 80
Insurance, 149–150
Integrated healthcare, 164
Internet of Things (IoT), 30, 165
Investments:
in 2020, 102
in digital healthcare, 64–65, 154–159
driving force for, 159

Invisibility of digital health, 4–5, 170
Invitae, 96
Invite Media, 92
IoT (Internet of Things), 30, 165

J

JD Health, 157
Jeong, Saeju, 127
Johnson & Johnson Innovation Labs (JLABS), 107

K

Kaia Health, 79
Kaiku Health, 76
Khorana, Har Bogid, 86
Kinect sensor, 22
Krein, Steven, 109–110

L

Lai, Matteo, 11–12
Large companies, strategy and politics of, 152
Lee, Stan, 136
Levy, Monique, 25–26
Life sciences companies, 170–171
Lifestyle as medicine, 121–130
Headspace, 125–126
HealthTunes, 126–127
Noom, 127
Pioppi Protocol, 128
Roberto's vision for, 123–125
from self-empowerment to, 122
Sleepio, 127–128
Werzowa on, 129–130
YourCoach.health, 81, 128
Lifestyle habits:
to manage blood pressure, 77–78
Omada Health's devices and curriculum for, 45
Livongo, 47, 57, 61–62

Loman, Nicholas, 87
Loose, Matthew, 87

M

Machine learning (ML), 17, 18, 89
Made of Genes, 97
Malhotra, Aseem, 128
Manic behavior, 79
Masimo, 109
MASK, 37
Massachusetts Institute of Technology (MIT), 10
Mass screening, big data in, 16–18
Materials, for processors and sensors, 4
Maxam, Allan, 86
Mayo Clinic, 42
Mazik Global, 158
Medical records, 18
Meditation, 125
Mediterranean Diet, 128
Mehl, Konstantin, 79
Melanoma, 23
Mendel, Gregor, 86
Mental health, 26, 38, 169
Mental illness, 9. See also specific conditions
Metabolomics, 88
Microbiomics, 88
Microsoft, 22, 36, 158
Microsoft Cloud for Healthcare, 158
Milburn, Kristin, 114–115
Mindfulness training, 125
MindMaze, 37
MindPlay, 37
Miniaturization, 4, 5
MinION, 87
MIT (Massachusetts Institute of Technology), 10
MIT Media Lab, 26, 79
Mixed reality, 36

ML, see Machine learning
Moonshot mission, 110
MSD Foundation, 108
Music, 122, 124, 126–127, 129–130
MusicMedicine, 129–130
MyHeritage, 96

N

Nanopore, 87
Nanotechnology, 4
Nanotechnology-based devices, 4
National health services, 152
National Institute for Infectious Diseases, Rome, 87
Network-connected devices, 4. See also Devices, sensors, and signals
Neurological diseases, 73
Neurostimulation, 10
Next-generation sequencing (NGS), 87–88
Ng, Andrew, 26
Nirenberg, Marshall W., 86
Noom, 127
Novartis, 74, 107, 109
Novartis Biome, 102, 107
Novo Nordisk, 127
Nueno, Carlos, 49–50
Nuro, 118
Nurses, robot, 31

O

Oak Street Health, 158
Observational healthcare, 163
Oleena, 80
Omada Health, 45
On-demand healthcare services, 43
One Drop, 20–21, 24–25
O'Neill, Donal, 128

One Medical, 158
Open Accelerator, 107–108
Open innovation and partnerships,
    99–120
  AlmirallShare, 103
  Bayer G4A, 21, 102, 104. *See also*
      Bayer G4A; G4A program;
      Grants4Apps
  Digital Garden, 103
  Dowe on, 112–113
  Estrella on, 118–119
  Frontiers Health, 104–105
  Healthware Labs and Healthware
      Life Hub, 105–106
  HealthXL, 106
  Johnson & Johnson Innova-
      tion Labs, 107
  Milburn on, 114–115
  Novartis Biome, 107
  Open Accelerator, 107–108
  Patients' Digital Health
      Awards, 108
  Pfizer Healthcare Hubs, 108
  Roberto's vision for, 101–103
  Roche HealthBuilders, 109
  Seuntjens on, 116–117
  speed and intuition of smaller
      companies, 100–101
  StartUp Health, 109–110
  Stoakes on, 111–112
  Vertical, 110–111
Open innovation model, 102
Otsuka, 9, 109
Outset Medical, 158
Oxford Nanopore, 87

P

Pacifica, 117
Page, Larry, 90
Paginemediche, 55–57, 62–63
Palomer, Xavier, 38

Pande, Vijay, 72
Panopticon, 30
Parkinson's, 126
Partnerships, *see* Open innovation
      and partnerships
PatchAi, 39
Patients:
  digital health ideas from
      perspective of, 108
  factors feeding distorted
      behavior of, 137
  future data collection and
      storage by, 148
  as healthcare consumers,
      135–138, 140
  health management by, 154
Patients' Digital Health Awards
      (PDHA), 108
Payment management, 61
Pear Therapeutics, 73
Pepper Robot, 37–38
Personal data, 6
  in medical records, 18
  patients' access to, 148–149
  and pervasive
      technologies, 30
  privacy of, 17
Personal genomics, 85–97
  Cellarity, 94–95
  Deep Genomics, 91–92
  evolution of genetics, 86–88
  Flatiron Health, 92–93
  Flores on, 95–97
  Human Longevity, 93–94
  Roberto's vision for, 88–90
  Sophia Genetics, 94
  23andMe, 90–91
Personalized health, 62
Personal medical devices, 1
Petakov, Artem, 127
Peter Munk Cardiac Centre, 7
Pfizer, 76, 77, 108
Pfizer Healthcare Hubs, 102, 108

Pharma:
   customer engagement by, 170–171
   telehealth approach of, 172
Physiotherapy, 79
Piedmont Healthcare, 55
Pierson, Rich, 125–126
Pills:
   with micro-sensors, 5, 8–9
   smart pill containers, 30
PillPack, 171
Ping An Group, 109
Pioppi Protocol, 128
Places of care, 54–55
Platforms, see Digital health
         enabling platforms
Politecnico, Milan, 31
Politics of healthcare
         sector, 153
Population growth, 152
Precision medicine, 93–94
Predictive data analysis, 148
Predictive data analytics, 48, 163
Prevention, big data in, 16–18
Preventive medicine, 163
Privacy:
   of data, 17, 148
   and pervasive
         technologies, 30
Production costs, 4, 5
Propeller, 73–74
Proteomics, 88
Proteus Digital
         Health, 4, 8–9
Psious, 38
Psoriasis, 10
Puddicombe, Andy, 125–126
Pushpala, Ashwin, 46

Q

Qardio, 9
Quasarmed, 77

R

Ramakrishnan, Shanti, 13–14
Randhava, Mohan, 58, 59
Razorfish, 24
Rehabilitation, 32, 37
Reimbursement management, 61
Relational agents, 25–26
Remote monitoring. See also
         Telemedicine and remote
         monitoring
   devices and technologies
         for, 44–45
   of network-connected
         devices, 4–5
   platforms for, 43
ResearchKit, 58–59
Revolutions in healthcare, 162–168
Risk of disease development, 91
Ro, 172
Robotics, 31–33
   domotics, 33
   Pepper Robot, 37–38
   in remote surgeries, 44–45
Robot nurses, 31
Roche, 109, 119
Roche HealthBuilders, 76,
         93, 102, 109
Rose, David, 30

S

Salesforce, 55
Sanger, Frederick, 86
Sanger method, 86
San Mateo Medical Center, 22
Sano, 46
Sanvello, 117
Schizophrenia, 78
Schrodinger, 158
SCOR, 21
Seattle Flu Study, 7

Seizure detection, 8
Self-service healthcare plans, 171
Sensely.com, 21–22
Sensors, 74. *See also* Devices,
　　sensors, and signals
SensorFusion, 48
Seuntjens, Steve, 116–117
Shuren, Jeffrey, 91
Sidekick Health, 76
Signals, *see* Devices, sensors,
　　and signals
Skin cancer, 23, 117
SkinVision, 23, 117
Slaughter, Mark, 59
Sleep improvement, 127–138
Sleepio, 72–73, 122, 127–128
Slujis, Marc, 63–65, 72
Smaller companies:
　　radical innovation by, 105–106.
　　　　See also Open innovation
　　　　and partnerships
　　speed and intuition of, 100–101
Smoking cessation, 78
Social networks, 54, 166. *See also*
　　Digital health
　　enabling platforms
Softbank Robotics, 37–38
Somyryst, 73
Sophia Genetics, 94
Speeches, by Roberto
　　Ascione, 175–176
Speech recognition, 32–34
StartUp Health, 43, 109–112
Stoakes, Unity, 110–112
Stress relief, 10
Symptom journal, 6

T

Taliossa, 119
Ted Rogers Centre for Heart
　　Research, 7

Teladoc Health, 46–47,
　　50, 57, 62
Tele-assistance, 42
Telehealth, 169
Telemedicine (in general):
　　barriers to, 43
　　during Covid-19 pandemic,
　　　　42, 44, 169
　　definitions of, 42
　　in Europe, 42–43
　　new tools developed for, 55–56.
　　　　See also Digital health
　　　　enabling platforms
Telemedicine and remote moni-
　　toring, 41–51
　　bringing a human face to, 21–22
　　Covid-19 and telehealth,
　　　　44, 154
　　life changes with, 42–43
　　Nueno on, 49–50
　　Omada Health, 45
　　Roberto's view on, 44–45
　　Sano, 46
　　Teladoc Health, 46–47, 50
　　TytoCare, 47–48
　　VitalConnect, 48
Tempus, 158
Tencent, 157
Thurner, Manuel, 79
Thync, 10
Training:
　　for the digital transformation,
　　　　143–144
　　of doctors, 144
Transformation of health care,
　　173. *See also* Digital
　　transformation of
　　healthcare
Trust, 147–150
Turner, Nat, 92
23andMe, 90–91, 95
TytoCare, 47–48

U

UCL (University College of
        London), 31, 126
UnitedHealthcare, 7
United Health Group, 117
University College of London
        (UCL), 31, 126
University Health Network, 7
University of California, Irvine, 7
University of Technology,
        Delft, 31
University of Washington School of
        Medicine, 7

V

Validation of digital health
        interventions, 139–140
Venter, Craig, 93
Venture Design, 104
Veritas Genomics, 96
Vertical, 110–111
Virta health, 73
Virtual reality (VR), 31, 32, 37, 38
VitalConnect, 48
Vitality, 66
Voice technologies, 32–34
Voluntis, 80
VR, see Virtual reality

W

Watson, James, 86
Wearables, 4, 6–7, 142. See
        also Devices, sensors,
        and signals
    Apple Watch, 6–7, 9
    Empatica
        smartwatch, 8, 12
    and insurance, 150
Weight loss, 45, 127
Weinberg, Zach, 92
Werzowa, Walter, 129–130
Woebot Health, 25–26
Wojcicki, Anne, 90
Worldwide investments
        in digital
        healthcare, 154–159
Wysa, 158

Y

YourCoach Health, 81, 128. See
        also Lifestyle as medicine;
        YourCoach.health

Z

Zcube (Zambon Research Venture),
        107